BEATING CANCER
WITH THE
HELP OF EINSTEIN

BEATING CANCER WITH THE HELP OF EINSTEIN

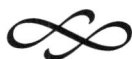

DONALD WOOD

Copyright © 2015 by Donald Wood.

Library of Congress Control Number: 2015900691
ISBN: Hardcover   978-1-5035-0156-0
         Softcover   978-1-5035-0155-3
         eBook   978-1-5035-0157-7

All rights reserved. No part of this book may be reproduced or transmitted in any form or by any means, electronic or mechanical, including photocopying, recording, or by any information storage and retrieval system, without permission in writing from the copyright owner.

Any people depicted in stock imagery provided by Thinkstock are models, and such images are being used for illustrative purposes only.
Certain stock imagery © Thinkstock.

In preparing this information, we have used our best endeavours to ensure that the information contained herein is true and accurate. We accept no responsibility and disclaim all liability in respect of any errors, inaccuracies, misstatements, website information, equipment used, their application, medications, and suggested remedies by way of this book.

Prospective purchasers should make their own assessment of the information provided and take steps to verify the information if they intend to rely on it.

Please note: Any exercise you do is at your own risk, and any information provided in this book is given "as is," without warranties of any kind, as we all vary. If you feel uncomfortable with any of the exercises mentioned, please talk to your personal physical trainer. If you have a serious disease, discuss this with your physician, who should consider these exercises in relation to the disease(s) you have and the success percentage rate of what the physician is offering as well as the possibility of blending the two factors: Western medicine and these exercises.

Print information available on the last page.

Rev. date: 03/30/2015

To order additional copies of this book, contact:
Xlibris
1-800-455-039
www.Xlibris.com.au
Orders@Xlibris.com.au

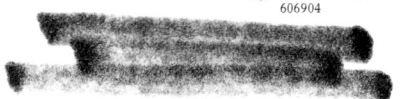

606904

Contents

1. Knowing Jean 17
2. Off to the Airport En Route to South America 22
3. Jean and the Guru 27
4. Jean Loses her Battle 34
5. Family Comparisons 37
6. Fulfilling My Promise–Travel and Research 42
   Bama, Guingui, and China 42
   Okinawa 55
   Shanghai to Urumqi, Hetian, Yutian, Layisu 73
   Islamabad, Pakistan 74
   Hotan, or Hetan, as it can be known 75
7. Western and Ancient Worlds 92
8. Static Electricity 99
9. Final Results–Electromagnetic Radiation 108
10. The Einstein Connection 110
    Understanding Personal Body Balance
    The First Line of Defence 114
11. Kirlian Photography 118

12. Understanding Meditation 122
13. Stress Proteins..128
14. Apartment Living...131
15. Daily Routines to Maintain Health 136
16. Bridget, Jason, Ben, and Don 143
17. Food and Diet...146
18. Exercise 149
19. Air Travel and Associated
    Problems and Possible Solutions................................151
20. Carcinogenic Products 159
21. Recommendations for the Building Industry..........163
22. Bacteria...167
23. Eliminating Bacteria..177
24. Recommendations and Solutions..............................188
25. A Miracle? Positive Verification 2013.......................194
26. Conclusion..208

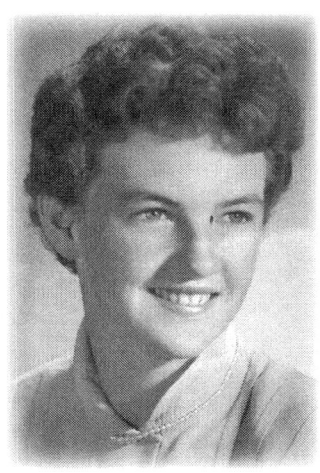

To my beautiful wife, Jean, who was taken away from me before we had fulfilled our adventures and dreams.

I promised her I would investigate as to why many pockets of the world have "long-livers" who are free from the dreadful disease of cancer and the like, and this book is proof of my efforts.

I hope that my research aids in the handling, treatment, and prevention of the spread of disease and in doing so may help to eradicate it all together.

INTRODUCTION

THIS BOOK RELATES a true story of two lovers, Jean and Don, who had been together since their early teens and who lived a brilliant, exciting, and interesting life. Then seemingly from nowhere, disaster struck when they were faced with the prospect of incurable cancer throwing their lives into trauma and financial difficulties, with death on any day a likelihood.

Many different avenues were followed in the search to extend Jean's life: pranic healing, healthily grown organic foods, getting back to nature frequently, and keeping her body grounded as much as possible to allow beneficial negative ions to flow through her body.

Don made a promise to Jean on her deathbed that he would travel the world and study why some people live well into their hundreds seemingly disease-free, while we in the Western world are succumbing to horrible and deadly diseases every day. His study led him to China, Okinawa, and so forth, seeking out the centenarians of the world, seeing how they live, what they eat, and drawing comparisons to friends and family.

The main elements that kept coming up were electrical body balance and grounding. The word grounding is the same as an electrician uses when referring to electricity in our households or businesses. Grounding in the electrical world means that the electricity has been allowed to go to Earth, thereby completing an electrical circuit. Our bodies are made up of skin, bones, blood, and so forth, as well as ions that flow through our bodies, grounding us to the earth. "Earthing" decreases the effects of potentially disruptive electronic fields. By being earthed and grounded, we improve our heart rates, inflammation, and nervous systems, also reducing stress. This book goes on to explain how we can maintain good negative body balance by eating healthy foods, exercising, meditation, and de-stressing, all of which helps us to fight disease. Don's theory is that the secret to longevity is in our living conditions—namely staying grounded and maintaining a good negative body balance.

Static is usually a man-made product that indicates that in a human being, his electrical balance is in imbalance. This imbalance can accumulate and reach dangerous levels. The normal balance is where there are equal positive and negative elements. Excessive amounts of positive can cause electric shocks and do not let the body perform naturally, as nature intended. This book explains various ways of bringing this static back to normal.

I thought there might be something in this static situation, as it is totally unnatural to have anything going around like this in our bodies.

The final chapters are based on areas that need attention in our society because they are responsible for breeding and spreading bacteria from one person to another. We have shown ways of sterilizing notes and cash to eliminate some of this spread of disease and have manufactured machines to cope with the problem.

It has been assessed that something like fifteen million people worldwide are likely to die within a year from various diseases, including cancer. We can all help ourselves to fight disease and live to one hundred or more.

As the medical profession is being constantly challenged, so will this book be, but due to the importance of the information contained herein to so many people trying to stay alive in good health, we want to convey the blow-by-blow descriptions of what we did to create what we and the medical profession referred to as a miracle by way of extending the life of our loved one. We have to get the message across. Discrepancies and many ways of upgrading or updating our findings will come along, but it is important to get the message across in order to help those with and without disease to begin having extended lives *today*!

The purpose of this book is to get this message out to as many people as I can, to give them extended life in good condition, as Jean had. This research will be left to others to pursue, as time is such an important factor for so many people.

Clarification of words used herein:

We are going to clarify some words used throughout this book. The term Winky, or Winky Shield, is used repeatedly and represents a counter-attack or a positive result towards the prevention of disease.

The name Winky originated from a nickname Jean had as a little girl, and out of respect for her internal fortitude in fighting off the inevitable, we used that "name" as our counter-attack.

Throughout the book, we divided the degree of seriousness of varying diseases, including cancer. Category one is for people who are in good health and who don't believe they require assistance. Category two is for people who are at risk because their health is in a serious situation, which may or not be fatal. Group three is for people with terminal illnesses. To a person who presents in any of these situations, the idea would be to use whatever they feel is necessary to bring themselves back into good health.

In everyday language, it offers explanations and solutions and sometimes inventions to those of us who are prepared to think outside the constantly daily indoctrinating medical square in which we have found ourselves.

ACKNOWLEDGEMENTS

ALBERT EINSTEIN; MASTER Danny; The University of Queensland; the World Health Organization; the interpreters and guides: Angel, Tamio, and Jilil; the centenarians; Professor Craig Wilcox, Katsu Yukama; Bryce Woodhouse; Bryce Wauchope; Peter Finlayson; Michael Patane; Peter Rochlin; Helen Watkinson; the Ballina Health Centre (nutritionists); Silvia Payton; Lilly Taylor; Andy Hayes; Corbis Corporation Australia and USA; Cameron Taylor; my family; and special thanks to Rae Walters

Should I have missed any of the wonderful people who have helped me put this information together, please accept this as my sincere thanks.

CHAPTER 1

Knowing Jean

THIS IS A story about my wife Jean, a most attractive woman. She was only five feet two inches in height and always strived to maintain a flat tummy and her fifty-five kilos. She lost an eye years ago, but her cosmetic artificial eye worked well.

I met Jean when I joined a local tennis club of which Jean was a member. You might say it was love at first sight. Jean was only fifteen years old then. She was such a live wire, full of fun, so outgoing and physically active. She used to laugh and refer to me as her "virgin."

She was always looking for the next competitive golf game, sailing race, event, or even parachuting army style. She was full of action, but she also gave strangers the impression that she was ladylike, well spoken, and well educated.

Like all married people, we had our difficulties sometimes, and I often thought that because of her volatility that had she had black hair instead of brown; she might have had some Italian blood in her. Together we were a volatile yet loving match, along with everything that goes with it.

When I was trying to start our business with no capital, Jean would take the children to school and use the vehicle to work as a courier to try to help balance the budget while I tried to make a success of my undercapitalized endeavours and inventions. She waited for years after our marriage before I could afford to buy her an engagement ring.

She was an outstanding sporting person, playing competitive tennis (that is, until she lost the eye) and golfing, playing pennants for her club. She particularly loved the golfing girls; they were so friendly and exciting, and every day was an adventure on the golf course.

Jean would do anything at all. We sailed many oceans together by yacht, did extensive travelling in Japan and the Arab world, and we even crossed Russia at the time of communism, when everybody was under suspicion. One time off eastern New Guinea, we encountered trouble when pirates boarded. We locked ourselves in the cabin as they tried to kick the cockpit door in, and Jean patiently kept practicing to reload the vary pistol (a mini rocket launcher), which was our only weapon. She followed instructions, and we worked together to fight them off and save the boat.

I remember how proud I was when we were caught in a storm yachting in the straits of Formosa. On that stormy night, we couldn't see the shore. We knew we were dangerously close, but we couldn't go into one of the most dangerous shipping channels in the world at night. Normally in a situation like that at sea, the rocks are what sink you. Sailing two up when I couldn't continue anymore because of exhaustion (with the yacht beating up the coast) and navigating off the chart's recorded depths and working off our depth sounder (which is a very risky business), she took the helm to give me a rest. For hours, she calmly beat head to wind in extreme seas until morning, when I could hold my own again and carry on. Daylight showed us a new cruise ship washed ashore, its layers of unused lifeboats sitting on the sky side of the ship on the beach. I was so proud of her efforts that I promised her a five-star meal ashore. However, when we got to the industrial port of Keelung, the best meal on offer was small pieces of bony fish wrapped in Taiwanese newspaper. We sat on blue milk crates picking off the newsprint from our fish. We had a domestic row there and then, with two security guards listening in!

She was, as you can gather, a champion sailor. She was also good on the trapeze, and in conjunction with her golfing, she did competitive regattas and had many championships under her belt. She received recognition in Canberra, Australia, for the never-to-be-repeated Bicentennial Medal for Excellence in Sport–Sailing. She modestly never spoke of her sailing achievements or the medal, which she kept in a drawer and which I proudly keep at home today.

Jean was a particularly caring person who easily made friends, and she sponsored many children around the world as well. Sadly, the first sponsored child died in the Vietnam conflict. Although it seemed like nothing to her, it was with great difficulty that she tried to get manually operated sewing machines to disadvantaged people in impossible places to help give them a lift and improve their lives.

All lives have their good and bad times, and probably one of the most disappointing times was when we were in Yemen on a holiday. An Australian had told us about a plant that he was convinced held healing powers and which could possibly help diabetes sufferers. In our efforts to locate this plant, we found ourselves in a minefield due to a civil war, and I don't have to tell you how terrifying that situation can be–too terrified to take a single step.

This success was never brought to bear due to the corruption at one end and impossible activities in Australia regarding the importation of vegetation at the other end, thus disappointing many people. This was when we ran into trouble health-wise, and our priorities, as you would expect, changed.

On the upside, of course, there was the time I sailed in beautiful smooth waters on a sea in Japan with my girl underneath my arm and snow-capped Mount Fuji ahead of us. There are magic moments, and there are disappointments. I will always remember those two things from our life together.

A funny story comes to mind. We were paddling down the Zambezi River in Zimbabwe, five two-man canoes and two other canoes carrying a single guide and provisions and a rifle. We were camping for the night in two-man tents along the shore, where there was Zambia on one side of the river and a giant nature reserve on the other, full of hippos, elephants, crocodiles, and so forth. In the darkness, we could see wild elephants right beside us, so the guides signalled with their torches—not trying to frighten them but trying to guide them away from our little camp of two-man tents. This woke me, and I wanted to go to the toilet. I told Jean that I was going to go behind the big termite mound, which was about twenty yards away.

I got to the other side of the termite nest and froze; I could hear something behind me. I quickly turned around. I had a toilet roll wrapped around a spade handle, which I carried for obvious reasons, and when I stopped, the noise stopped! My heart pounding, I went a little farther, and I realized I was being stalked. I whirled around, prepared to defend myself with my weapon—the dunny (an Aussie slang name for a toilet) spade—and discovered what was happening: the toilet roll had unwound as I walked along, and of course it stopped when I stopped. *I was being stalked by a toilet roll!* Life was fantastic.

CHAPTER 2

Off to the Airport En Route to South America

WE HAD PLANNED a holiday to South America, and we patiently sat at the Sydney airport in Australia, waiting for our flight via Air Argentina. We were so excited, as we had never been to South America except for going around it once by cruise ship when we circumnavigated the island of Cape Horn for what we thought then would possibly be our last opportunity to tackle Cape Horn via sailing boat–examining areas for possible refuge in case of storms.

Jean left for a moment to phone our daughters–we have four, two of whom were running the family business–and then we got our final boarding call and hopped on the plane. We flew economy/coach class, as we always did, and settled in for what was expected to be a pleasant flight, with only one stop in New Zealand, about three hours out of Sydney.

The plane seemed nice, and the service was good. All of a sudden, Jean said, "I don't feel well at all." I asked her what was the matter, and she replied, "I don't know, but I feel dreadful." I called the chief steward—his name was Peter—a very competent man. She was almost unconscious as she said, "I am in dreadful agony."

"Is there a doctor on board?" we heard over the loudspeaker. Here we had a person who seldom got sick, hardly ever got the flu, and three doctors came forward on the plane. The plane was full, and they moved her into upper class, where she could be more comfortable.

The doctors went to ask for the medical kit on the plane, but unfortunately, all the kits on the plane were in Spanish; that was not good news. There was an ambulance waiting for her at Auckland, and she was rushed to the hospital.

The New Zealand hospital was excellent, and the service was good. They were probably as good as you could get in any area of the world—and with probably more attention. After a short period of time the unfortunate diagnosis came: she had liver cancer. The cancer was a melanoma as big as a fist on the liver itself, which she had known nothing about. The message was that if we could get her back to Australia, they still could not be sure if the immediate problem could be stopped from spreading. She would be lucky if she had three months to live, and she would have to look at life on a daily basis.

I don't have to tell you the shock, not only for her but also for the entire family. This sort of thing happens to other people and just does not happen to people who are so adventurous, seemingly healthy, and apparently strong. I was seventy-six years old, and Jean was seventy-four. We had been married forty-six years. Jean was diagnosed in mid-2005.

After returning to Sydney, we went to a specialist who was possibly the best in the world. We were prepared to travel anywhere, but unfortunately, the diagnosis came up the same in every instance. When asked point-blank if she really had only three months to live (You almost had to hold a gun to the doctor's head to get a truthful answer), we were told that she would be lucky to get that. However, they said she could try chemotherapy. The extension of life by chemo might be only a couple of weeks and knowing how sick it can make you, she elected not to have it. The dosage would have been massive, and it tends to kill everything. As it turned out, it was a fateful decision.

The first action in New Zealand was morphine to stop the pain, and this had an adverse effect on her and aggravated the problem. There was nothing the medical profession could do for us anywhere in the world—money was no object, and we were prepared to pay anything, but money could not solve this problem, and when we found out that liver cancer is one of the most agonizing of all deaths, it created panic in both of our minds.

When asking the doctors about this, explaining that morphine had a bad effect, they said they would find something else when the time came. Of course, we were not happy about that. She could be part of an experiment in agony when that time arose. We'd heard of a euthanasia organization, and we contacted them, saying that we would want to be able to terminate her life when she couldn't stand the pain anymore. Because of laws in Australia making euthanasia illegal, they could not say they advocated euthanasia; however, they described to us how we could go about it, but it would have to be her own choice, of course. When they gave us this information, it was like a giant load had being lifted off Jean. You could see the change in her once she knew that she could take control of things and prevent herself from having an agonising death. I might add that we did not easily make these decisions. Every decision is somewhat fatalistic and wanting reassurance at all times.

We got involved with this Queensland (a northern state of Australia) euthanasia organisation as far as we could. They later moved to Darwin (Australian Northern Territory). Jean was totally relieved. They never wanted any money and never asked for anything. It was all a matter of trying to help someone have a pleasant death if it became necessary. Who knew what the future could hold. In life, circumstances change and new medications become available.

We heard of a doctor in Ballina, which is approximately four hundred miles north of Sydney, a naturopath who was into alternate medicines. We got involved with great volumes of vitamins after finding out that there were no adverse effects with any particular vitamins (which can happen if one is pregnant, for instance). They recommended a United States organization making very powerful health tablets, and she had direct infusions of vitamin C. These two things seemed to help for a while. We eventually cut the vitamin C out when we felt it was not helping.

We also had a compound tablet made up to be placed between the cheek and gum—one troche only—if feeling ill or unwell.

CHAPTER 3

Jean and the Guru

JEAN HAD BEEN out of the hospital for approximately one month when an interesting thing happened: she started visually ageing. My daughter is involved in alternate medicines, crystals, and a type of healing called pranic healing. Pranic healing is a simple yet powerful system of no-touch energy healing, mainly used to create energy within the body with the use of crystals. She is very much into this alternative lifestyle, which is very diverse to a person like myself. It is hard to get your head around something that is not part of our Western way. She was informed that her guru doctor, Master Danny, was coming to give a lecture in the town hall Sydney suburb of Mosman, which is quite close to where we lived, to try to get more people involved in this type of medicine. He agreed to try his methods of healing on Jean but pointed out at the time, even before his lecture to a packed audience, that he could not cure cancer.

After the lecture was over—and after receiving a good reception from everybody—this smartly dressed amicable chap who appeared to be in his forties decided to have a look at Jean. He suggested we go to the little room at the side of the vestibule of the town hall. He asked that we bring a bowl of salted water with us. He asked Jean to sit down, and he began to wave crystals at her. You can imagine what we thought, being brainwashed in the principals of conventional Western medicine. You the reader are probably also thinking that this is a bit on the way-out side.

This went on for about a half hour, and he produced a white handkerchief from time to time. He moved himself around her whilst she sat in the chair. He waved crystals over several parts of her body and then wiped the crystals with the handkerchief and held it over the salted water—thus giving the impressing that he had gathered the impurities from her body on the crystals and was then putting them into the salted water. At no time was her body touched by the crystals or by the handkerchief. All this was done with very serious concentration.

This went on in the front of her mostly, finally finishing off by waving the crystals down the back of her. When he finished, he said, "Now you are going to get a result from this, and it will be almost immediate." Personally, I found this a bit hard to swallow. He said to go straight home. It was the weekend, and he said that on Thursday she would feel a lot better. He reiterated that he couldn't cure cancer but said this would help in the interim. He was very confident that we would get some sort of reaction.

When we came home, Jean rushed to the entrance of the house and proceeded straight to the toilet. She experienced a large bowel movement, which was unexpected because she thought her bowels were working at normal levels. On Thursday morning, she woke up and said, "I think that I will go have a game of golf today." Now remember that this was a person dying of cancer—we were actually witnessing her die. We could not understand it, and we thanked our daughter, of course, and sent Master Danny a note thanking him as well, saying it was a very favourable result. We still could not get our minds around the new situation.

My mind was taken back to when I was a boy. My mum, who died at almost 104, made us take a dose of Epsom salts once a month. I am sure many of you remember this old-fashioned remedy. The family would cringe at the thought of taking this "medication," which tasted so dreadful and left us with diarrhoea. We had to hold our noses and take two or three great gulps of this awful mixture that had been dissolved in warm water. We would follow this with an orange or something sweet to rid ourselves of the taste. Within a very short time, we were racing to the toilet, and the smell was horrific! This smell had come from our body waste, and it may have been there for weeks. Your body would be left cleansed, free from rubbish, poisons, and maybe bacteria. You may wish to talk to your doctor about this logic, but I am sure you would instead be prescribed a mixture or tablet that didn't taste too bad and had the same reaction.

We got in touch with the guru in the Philippines and suggested that perhaps we might move to the Philippines, but he again emphasized that he could not cure cancer and suggested that we talk to his followers of the pranic style of healing. We tried many of them but did not feel that we were getting anywhere. My daughter appeared to be better than anyone else we had found in that regard.

It had been three weeks now since the prognosis of only three months to live. Life almost returned to normal, and we concentrated on good food (which she always ate) and exercise. Contrary to what the doctors were saying in relation to the fact that morphine and other things could be used, we pointed out that morphine in New Zealand had a bad effect, aggravating the problem.

We didn't think a lot about the *cancer*. Jean was playing good golf and concentrating on the garden. It gave her pleasure to be digging, picking up tools, and sweeping the leaves, which were always a problem in the area where we lived. The family visited her daily—no family frustration or worries, no being morbid, no stress. Everything was good. Sex life was normal. She was physically doing a lot of work, not sitting back on her backside waiting to die.

Over 5 years plus since the cancer was diagnosed we heard of a research group at a Queensland University that was having some success with a program that provided what we thought was a nonintrusive treatment (apart from taking medicine about once every couple of weeks). Jean elected to get involved in the program that applied to people who were terminally ill. Jean was showing quite good health at this particular time, and we both thought that this would probably not do her any harm. We would fly up to Brisbane every couple of weeks and do what was necessary. After about a month or two of this—I am going from memory here—when Jean came out of the hospital one time, I asked her how it went. She replied, "Good." As we were driving along, I was surprised that she was so quiet. She said they had changed the dosage of the chemo, and we hadn't even realised that the treatment she was being given actually included chemo, and what's more, this was to be her last session. Now I stopped the car—you have to realize that we were always in each other's mind. We vowed that we would not touch chemo, as it seemed so stupid to poison the rest of your body by using this treatment.

This was a big mistake, for now the very thought of chemo stressed us out completely. We had been thinking positively all the time. Everything we had done was without stress. Life had been happy. We talked about death as though it were a game of football. It was not like the end of the world—yes, it was the end of her life, but the misery of what was going to happen to her on the way to her death was what concerned us. She needed reassurance. We had thought all along that chemo was not the way to go, and here we were now, with Jean already having had several sessions.

We needed to have positive thinking to reinforce our minds that we were on the right track—the right program personally to defeat that disease. If you believe in something strongly enough, you will fight for what you believe and hopefully conquer it, making yourself happier in your own mind. For instance, you could have read somewhere that if you wear jade on your left wrist it will have a positive effect. So if you wear a jade bracelet and put positive faith in that bracelet, it gives you a reassuring lift. After all, the Chinese list jade in their medical library, as they consider it a mineral medicine. All of the people who wear jade seem to have this ability to defeat disease. We understand that when jade is worn close to the body, it creates a chemical reaction.

You have to believe that it works. You have to believe you are doing the right thing, and in turn your body will believe it too. An interesting investigation would be to evaluate the people who aren't doing well with these diseases and find a way of convincing them that they are going to be better off by doing what they are doing. It does not have to be jade; it can be anything. Shoes could be examined to make sure that they are not rubber soled but are of a type of construction to allow the beneficial negative ions to pass through to the ground, thereby making you grounded. It could be something that you possibly believe may give your body a lift. We are using the word Winky as your counter-attack–your ability to create positive thinking.

Jean had particularly strong ideas about health prior to her disease, and one thing that she would never have was air conditioning in the house. She loved her garden, and as you will see from the photograph of the garden, she had big trees you could hardly wrap your arms around. She had rows of camellias up to about twelve feet high. You couldn't work in the garden and not be totally grounded due to the vegetation. You couldn't go from one section of the property to the other because local laws governing swimming pools meant that the pool had to be isolated from the rest of the garden or yard with a self closing gate and safety fence. We only had one gate for safety reasons and this was situated near the back door of the house. These fences and gates were made of steel, which meant Jean would be grounded whenever she came into contact with them.

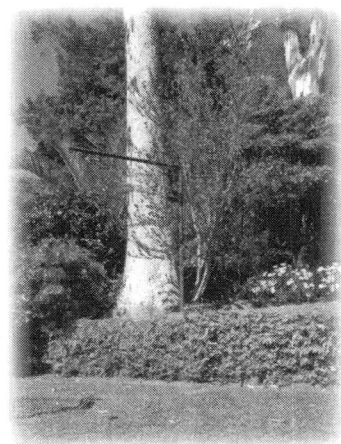
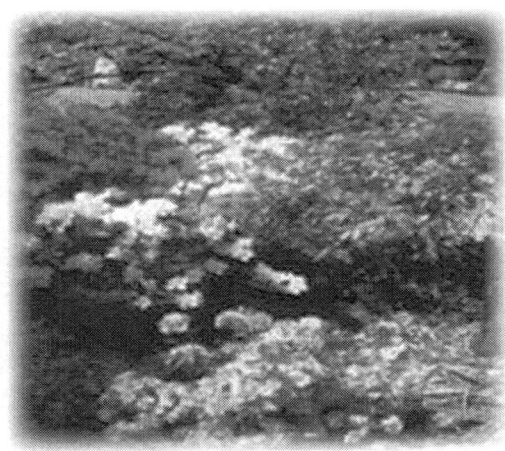

Jean's garden

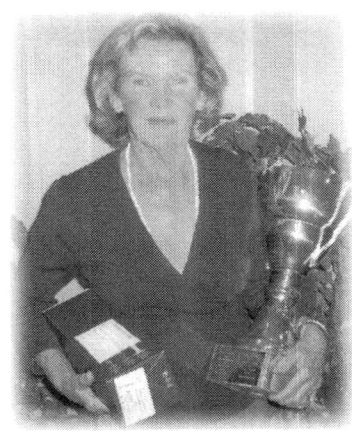
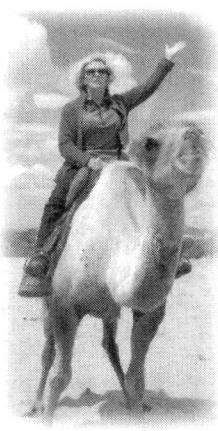
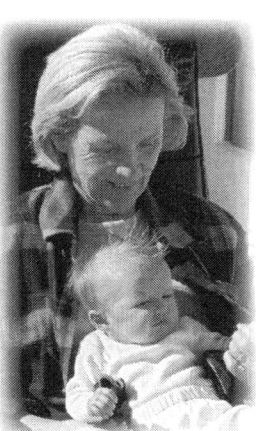

From the album

CHAPTER 4

Jean Loses her Battle

AFTER GOING TO a marvellous birthday party with close friends some five and a half years after being carted off the aeroplane at Auckland, and after many discussions between Jean and myself about what I was going to do when she left the stage, I decided that I was going to find out how we managed to pull off such a miracle. I would get some muscle in the form of guards and research the Arab world, particularly the Hunza area, where extended life seems to be the norm. Maybe we could do something to help people who were in serious trouble.

When we came home from the party that late afternoon, she was in good spirits, but during the night, her stomach swelled up; you would think she was four months pregnant. I rushed her to the hospital. They said there was nothing they could do, and by lunchtime the following day, I had lost my girl. Death happened quickly.

We had been planning new exciting adventures and enjoying parties with our good friends, and you could say that life didn't get any better. There was plenty of action going on, and we did not think about her illness or death ... and now she was gone. She had five years and three months or longer. Remember the original prognosis of three months maximum; she was prepared to die on a daily basis. Living that incredible percentage of over 2,000 per cent longer was a shock to everybody, including the doctors, who described it as a total miracle.

I was shattered and am still shattered at the loss. I thought about the plants we placed around our house and the gardening Jean did so she was earthed. The plants around the van my mum lived in were placed in a position to stop Mum from walking into the tow bar section, and these helped to ground the van. I had a flashback to so many years ago when I had the possibility of serious losses in business because of the machines giving off electric shocks, and how those people who touched those plants there became grounded. I said to my daughters who run the company, "There might be something in this earthing business, keeping your body in normal electrical balance to allow you to fight off diseases naturally." They replied, "Whatever you think, Dad," not taking much notice of it until I said that thought I would go see these oldies—the centenarians.

The family was extremely sympathetic about my loss at that particular time but asked why I wanted to do this. I told my four daughters that there would be something wrong with me if there was an opportunity for me to help people and I didn't do anything about it! I concede that it was a one hundred to one chance, but there was nothing to lose and everything to gain. I knew the chances were remote and the only figures that I had were that the average person, local or Western, carries about forty volts in his body as an average. We should keep open minds, discount the medical world, and look at this idea as a matter of physics—the idea being that if you have no static, you live a long life.

I had a personal static measuring machine flown out from America, which would give me the right answers as to the voltage carried by those ancient ethnic people. I worked on a principal that if they lived trouble-free and disease-free lives, then they were going to live for a long time. There is only limited and vague information known about their lifestyles, so I decided, to the surprise of all, to pack my bags, and off I went!

However, not being a young man, it first took me three months to get physically fit in addition to getting the equipment. But I considered my promise to Jean—that I would try to solve that problem—and that is what this book is all about.

CHAPTER 5

Family Comparisons

MY MUM DIED soon after Jean, just missing her 104th birthday by a matter of days–rarely sick in her whole life. It became my responsibility to dispose of my mum's home, a large aluminium mobile van/house that she had lived in for approximately twenty years. Upon examination of the van, I saw that the plumbing went to the ground, the electricity was earthing the van, and the two back tyres were deflated so you could barely see them because they had sunken into the earth. I realized that she would have been totally grounded all the time, meaning that as the van was earthed, her body was in electrical balance. The van was old, so any fumes from glues and so forth that were used in its construction would have dissipated long ago. Mum had such a disease-free long life.

The timber home that my wife loved so much was built in 1905 and rebuilt between the 1930s and 1940s, and it too would have been free from any building toxins. Jean would not allow any building additions to the house. She had an acceptable lifestyle once the guru from the Philippines got her back to normal.

We talked to the doctors to try to draw a comparison between Mum's life and that of Jean's. My theory was that we all need to be grounded. We need to have a balance of positive and negative ions to give the natural body balance, which we were created to have constantly. An example of an incorrect personal situation would be static electricity throwing your body into electrical turmoil. It was then that I realized that the only way to prove my theories and satisfy my mind was to research and talk to the long-livers in different parts of the world–people who live well into their hundreds in good health and are predominately disease-free.

As fate would have it, going back twenty-five to thirty years prior to that, I had an upsetting incident in my business career. A situation existed where machines were being changed from mechanical to electronic. Not everyone is proficient or familiar with electronics, so an unexpected market arose for those who could still supply these mechanical machines, and my company was perhaps one of the last or even the last that could supply them. I had a ready-made business.

One day I got a telephone call from a customer complaining that he or she was getting electric shocks from my mechanical equipment. Now, you cannot sell equipment that gives off electric shocks, so my old mechanic, Ralph, and I went urgently across the Spit Bridge, a suburb of northern Sydney, Australia. I can tell you that for a fellow who has been around, I was very shaky, for if I could not solve the problem of the machines giving off electrical shocks, I would be in a financial mess. I had committed myself to a full overseas factory production.

When we got over there, I found out that only one of the lasses in the organization of about seven was getting these shocks. I asked to see her—and no doubt about it: she touched the equipment and jumped, but the person who actually made the complaint was a customer who, by coincidence—or call it luck, if you like—came into the store at this particular time. I said, "Let's see you get a shock from this machine." When I had touched it, nothing happened, yet he nearly jumped through the roof. He was genuine in his reaction; it was nothing like the little lass from our organisation who got the first shock. Ralph said, "I can fix this," and I wondered how.

My heart was pounding. I could see a financial disaster looming in front of me. Ralph said, "Wait here for a few minutes." About ten minutes later, he came back through the doors of the shop with two large potted plants, and I thought, *What is he doing!* He said, "You owe me eighty dollars" (in today's money value). I said, "OK, what's going to happen now?" He put one of these plants, a fern, near the front door of the shop so that one would brush against it when entering the shop and another near the machine that was giving off the shocks. He told the fellow who complained to brush past the plant and then touch the machine. "What has happened," said Ralph, "is that the machine is not giving off the shocks; you are. It's called static electricity." I had never heard about that sort of a situation. Since the problem could be solved, I went on to create my first commercial real estate complex.

Static electricity within the body is an imbalance of ions—we should all aim to have a negative body balance. Too many positive ions create static electricity in our bodies, which is not good, as they are a primary cause of many major health problems. With the body being in an unbalanced state, it becomes vulnerable to any disease. As all diseases are caused through viruses and bacteria, an unbalanced body has no form of defence.

I don't have to tell you that the relief was profound. It was such a relief that I never forgot it. In those days, we did not have computers to be able to research this sort of static reaction.

I was obviously a busy man back then, but I heard—and it has to be classified as *hearsay* (a funny thing to resort to hearsay to describe these events that are going to change people's lives) of a fellow yachtsman who wanted to sail around Australia with his mates. He had leukaemia and went against medical advice. When he came back about a year later, he was free of the disease. No one could understand it. It was just one of those miracles that can happen, and it was sort of brushed aside as misdiagnosis, which is so common in the medical world in relation to things that cannot be explained.

We should point out here what static electricity actually is. Good electricity is live electricity that has current and is useful. Static electricity is also live electricity, but it does not have current. It is useless, and apart from electrical storms, it is unusual to have anything to do with the human body. However, this is not the case in this world we live in.

CHAPTER 6

Fulfilling My Promise—Travel and Research

Bama, Guingui, and China

THE PLACES I selected were those areas of the world that were recommended by the World Health Organization, where people are confirmed to be over one hundred years old.

The first place that I decided to visit was Bama in China, which is west of Nanning, in the south-western part of the country. The Okinawa's are a race on their own, occupied by the Japanese over the centuries. These areas were remote, away from civilization and the smog of big cities. Here I hoped to examine the centenarians and their way of life. I could study these people who lived without all the modern conveniences of the Western world, ate off the land, and who lived with nature. I hoped to be able to measure the electrical ions within their bodies and compare them to those of us who live in big cities. In fact, I hoped to find the secret of longevity.

The people from Bama are different from the Japanese. I thought that perhaps I would next have to go to the south west of China, to what turned out to be the Arab-like ethnic group of the west of China. If I continued at that particular point, I could go to the Hunzas of Pakistan, who are very well documented.

I was aware that the biggest problem that I would have (due to the fact there was no English spoken in these areas) would be language, and this prevented it from turning into a holiday. I thought that by using the upper-class hotels, I might solve this language problem, however. I got the concierges and managers to help me on arrival in Guangzhou, the old city of Canton. I went to a good four-star hotel, ringing up first and asking if there was anyone who could speak English. I was told that the manager spoke English, so I booked in. It turned out to be very good. I got all the detailed directions written down in both Chinese and English.

I needed to get to a city called Nanning, and from there I could jump off to the area of Bama. From Nanning, the manager referred me to his branch and to the right English-speaking connections. So I was doing pretty well, and within five days, I was actually in Bama.

It was quite a modern town by Chinese standards, very progressive, catering to all races but principally

Chinese. I had a wonderful stay. I met the Chinese guide who was organized by the hotel, and her name was Angel, an attractive and professional young lady. She took me out on the town, and we had a nice meal. It was a pleasant occasion and a quite enjoyable experience. The next day, we hopped in a car on a dirt road to a little village, and we stopped on the side of the road to read a sign: "Meet the old people of the world."

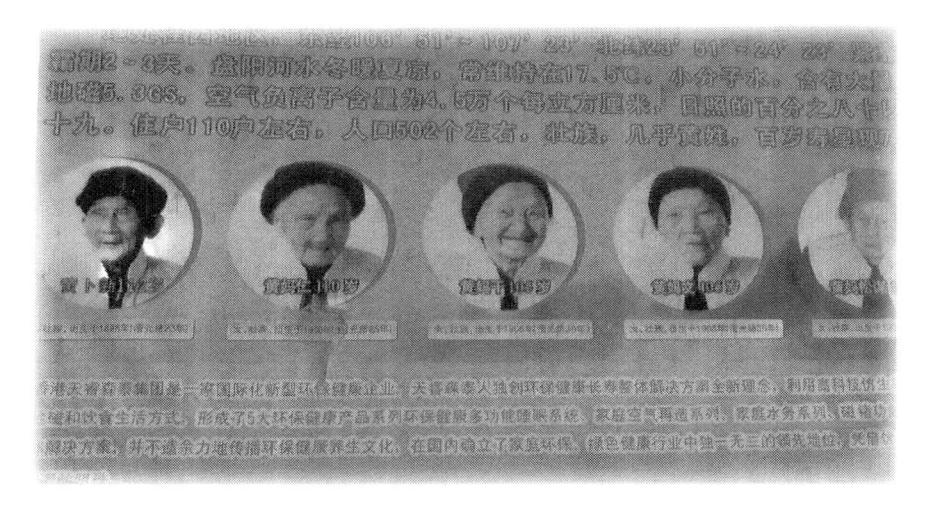

Meet the old people of the world

There were seven people who were over one hundred years old living in an area of about two hundred yards. It was at the bottom of the hill, coming down to the water's edge of a river that was fed by the lake behind it. The water was clear, and between the main road and us was a magnificent vegetable garden at the back, where the hills came down into the lake with a fine mist on the top.

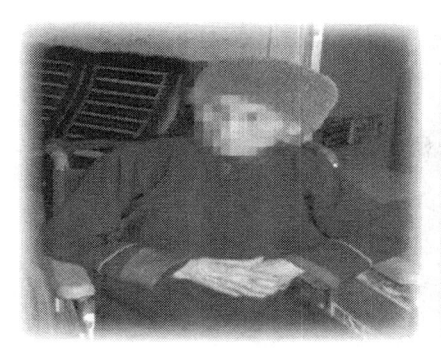

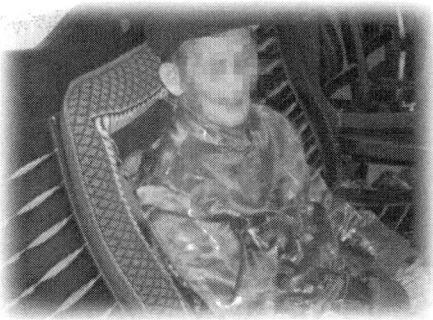

Some of the old people

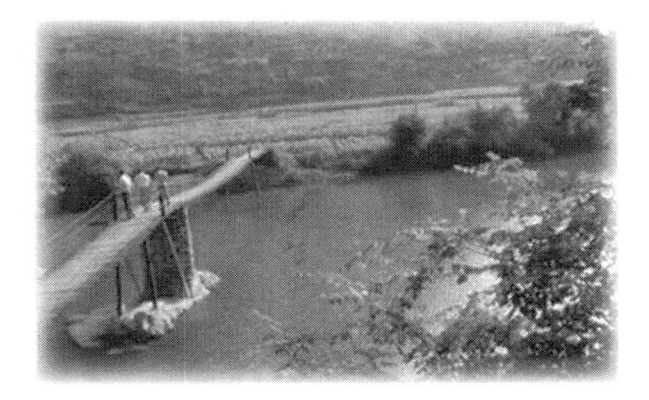

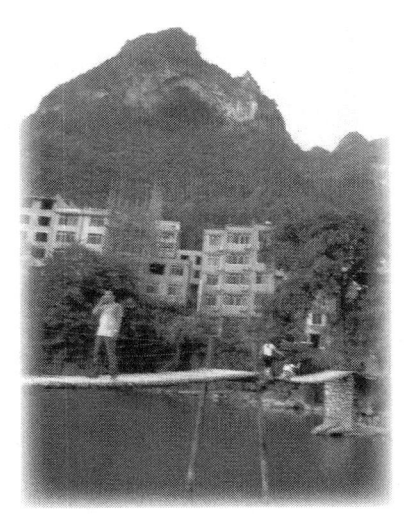

The town of Bama

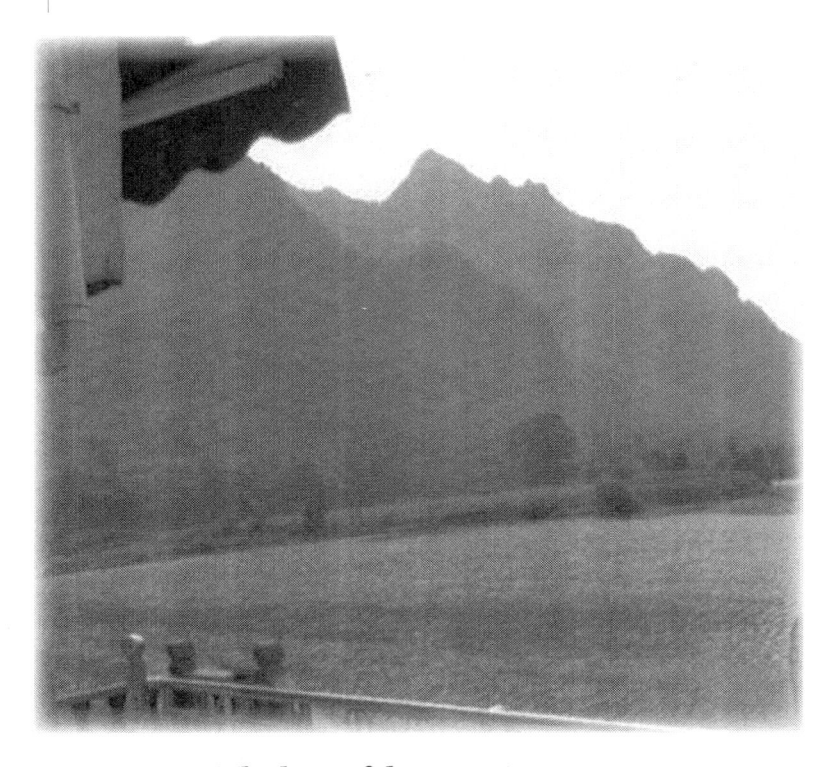

The beautiful mountain scenery

The scene was just like what you see Chinese artists draw. It was a beautiful, magical scene and a lovely place to enjoy. There was a causeway from the main road across a rough dirt road, bypassing many of the beautiful vegetable gardens. I say vegetables, but they call them herbs. In that area of the town, the buildings were built of old cement. They looked as though they might have been one hundred years old, nothing attractive about them at all. The insides of them were usually timber or cement with rugs.

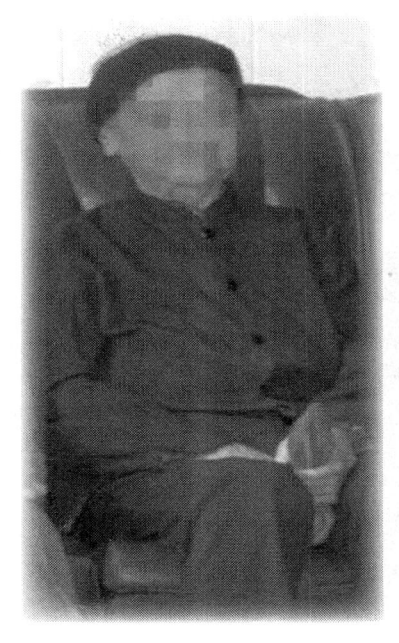

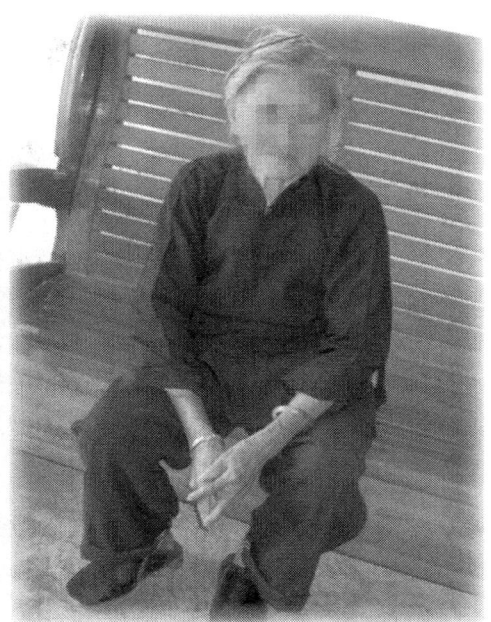

One of the "old people" clutching her red envelope

Note bracelets on both arms

We proceeded to talk to these people through the interpreter, Angel. They were very friendly and nice. They did not like to ask for money but would supply you with a little red envelope, and if you wanted to, you could leave them with a donation. Of course, everybody did, and they would say thank you and allow you to take a photo with them. They were happy to have some interest taken in them, and they readily consented and were often excited at being measured, unable to wait to hear the results. See the photo above. It was all so amicable, things were going according to expectations, and to my shock, we were getting no registrations of static at all. The averages were nothing like the forty volts we are supposed to get in the Western world–they were zero or close to it.

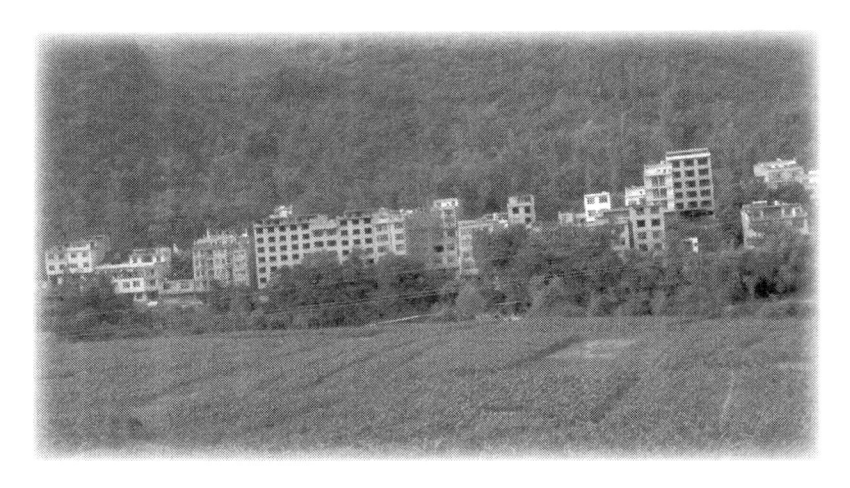

Centenarian village

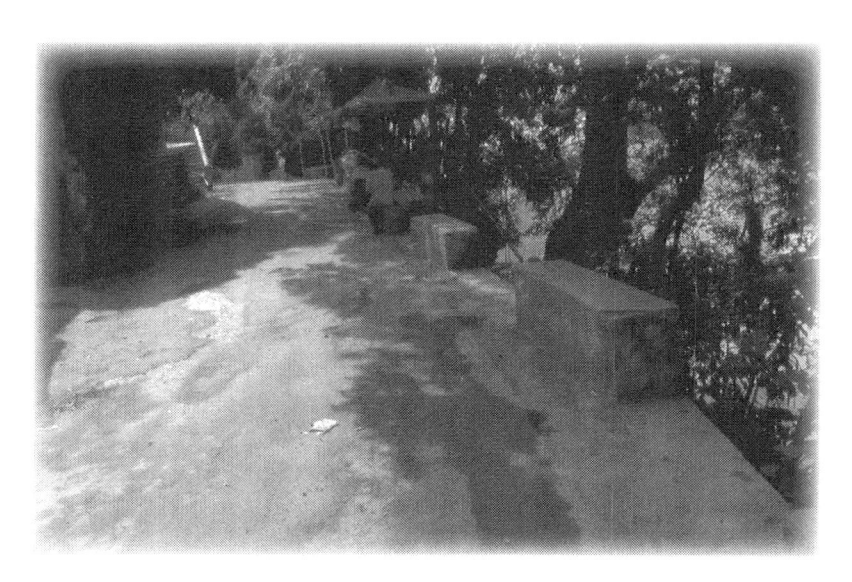

Main road

We came towards the end of that road, which was less than three hundred yards long, and we came across another woman who was in a slightly more modern brick building. Angel said it was OK to invite ourselves in. She was sitting on a little stool like a small child would use, but it did have a back on it. There were no cushions or anything like the other locations along the road, where people sat in old lounges, but they were still very comfortably catered for. I asked this woman, who was obviously rather old (she was one of those recognized as over one hundred), if I could test for static electricity. I always put the static measuring machine on myself first, both for grounding and to show that there were no shocks. The readings on the machine were extraordinary.

There were figures jumping everywhere for hundreds of volts, then down to 60 and back to 150, and then down to 30 and up to another 130. I could not understand what was happening. I went outside and saw power lines running along the edge of the river. All their homes were attached to them. These power lines were actually attached to the building that she was in, and I immediately concluded that these power lines had caused the wild electrical result. The woman was alive with bad electricity. I started to wonder how this could be, how she could still be alive if static was the problem. I could only assume that by her gardening, she was constantly grounded and that she had built up some sort of immunity. Then I learned that this woman actually lived on the hill, and to make things easier for her potential customers, she moved to this "alive house," which was on the level.

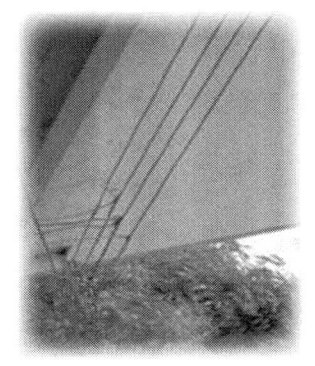

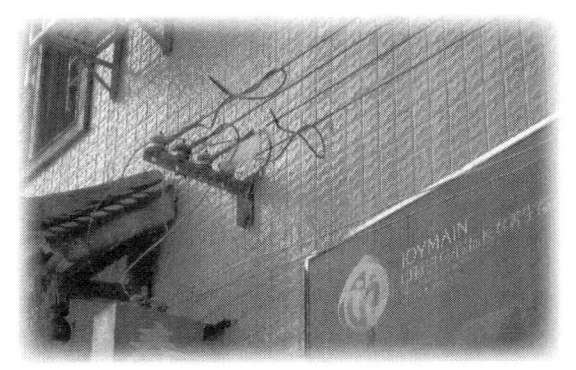

Power lines

Angel and I left her at this stage to see another woman up the hill. It was a steep hill but only about thirty yards long. It had bad steps and was quite awkward to get to. When we met this woman, she was grateful to see us. She was sitting on a hard uncomfortable seat, and I asked if I could check her electrical balance. She held out her hand after seeing me do it on myself, and she came up with zero static. I thought that was good because that was close to what the rest of town was, except for the woman down the bottom of the hill from her.

All the women had jade bracelets on their left wrists. On this woman's other hand, she had a silver bracelet, and I asked if I could measure her other hand, as I was interested in seeing what effect that would have on the machine. And to our surprise, it came up as nine volts! This turned out to be a key to the success of the overall venture. Wherever there was metal, it attracted electricity to the metal area on her body and removed the static from her body's critical areas, including the brain and so on.

It surprised me to see all these people wearing jade bracelets. In the city, you didn't see much jade.

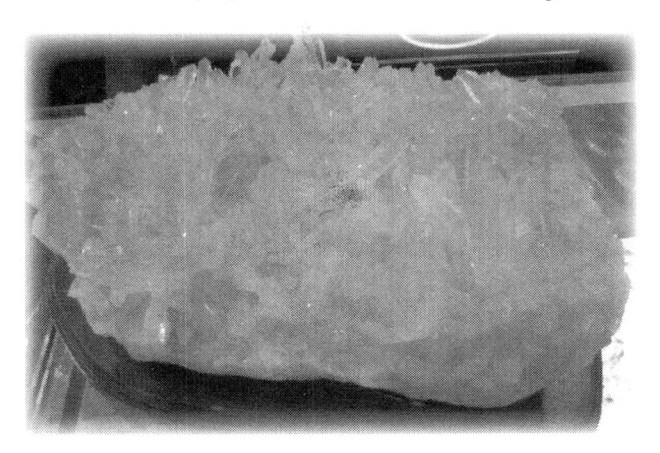

Crystals in hotel lobbies

At the motel that night, I tried to analyse what had happened. I realized how important the feature of the metal attraction capacity is and both how good and how bad it could be. With a long way to go still, I could not help thinking how dangerous it could have been had the woman been wearing metal-rimmed spectacles or if she had a metal hair clip that would attract the static into the brain area! On the other hand, by using this method, perhaps we could keep static away from dangerous areas of the body. Again, we had just started the personal survey and had a long way to go to see if this information would be useful or not.

There was often a big rock in the middle of the hotel lobbies along the way, and when you looked into it, you'd see that it was full of crystals—not necessarily jade. Not since the episode with the guru from the Philippines, who performed a shocking result with crystals, had anyone even mentioned crystals, except for my daughter, who, as I have said, is into this pranic healing. She actually has crystals on both sides of her workstation.

I tried to understand what was happening. Doing the reading of the electrical balance with my machine, I found that in the averages of all these people, it worked out that if I deleted the lowest, which would be a zero, and the highest and then did an average of the rest of the group, I could get a better average of the overall picture of the group. We needed to have an electrical body balance reading to compare with that of the Western world. I decided to do this in all the other locations I intended to go to and didn't use it unless numbers were too short to justify that theory.

The final electronic results of Bama: I excluded the woman who was running at 240-odd volts and jumping all over the place, which we believe was caused by the attachment of the house to the power lines and the relay systems that were associated to it (see photograph). If we deleted the highest and lowest of the group as a combined group of people and we got 2.5 volts. If we included all of the people and divided them by the number of persons, we got .5 of a volt. Now, allowing for the inaccuracy of the machine, which is under 2 volts, you could safely say that there was no dangerous electricity in any of the participants at all, except for the one woman on the stool.

As a matter of interest, the vegetables they ate were always very fresh, and there is reason to believe that the fresher the vegetables, the more beneficial they are to you.

This will be verified when we examine the information regarding health in the chapter on Kirlian photography; we can actually prove that this is correct.

We also should point out that the general consensus is that most of these people were usually vegetarians, and when this was not the case, they had fast little pigs about the size of a large cat, which they claimed were virtually fat-free when cooked. Also, they eat chickens and catch fish that are a small species of fish. They grow their own items and process their own food such as sugar, but they don't eat a lot of sugar, nor do they eat processed food. We should also mention here that they only generally eat what they have grown themselves. They have no stores in the village.

There was no doubt about the ages of these people as I compared them to the similar age of my mother about two years before she died, which would put them in the same vintage. I was told that in the year 2000, there were seventy-four centenarians in a population of 238,000 in the Bama region. An interesting viewpoint that came out of Angel's interpretation when trying to explain the balance of positive and negative is that they referred to it as yin and yang, their interpretation of body balance, which is exactly what we are talking about. It seems that they are some thousands of years ahead of us. They also related the words yin and yang to their chi when trying to clarify their interpretation of chi—the closest I could get to it was their energy resources.

The word energy keeps coming up, which, again, is what we are talking about. After having gone back the second day to clarify the readings where the electricity was in turmoil, the situation had divided itself in about half. The figures were still jumping all over the place, and they were nothing like they should be. I put this down to the fact that the power lines were the cause of the problem, and the power usage in the village that day may have been less than when the readings were taken previously. To me, this proves that electricity is creating problems with our health.

Angel looked after me, getting me back to the airport. I thanked her for doing an excellent job. I looked after her financially and got her to sign my report, which I did, of course, with all the guides.

I started to realize that going back in history and time, yin and yang was probably hundreds of years before electricity was actually invented. It wasn't until I was on the plane and had spoken to Angel that I realized that all the houses conformed to the basic principles of feng shui, facing south to catch the sun and having big open areas and plenty of trees, which, as mentioned, is necessary, even to the point of painting trees on the walls of their homes if they didn't have real trees around them.

(a) No one was over weight
(b) All ate about half of what we would eat
(c) No processed food available
(d) No commercial shop
(e) Food was super fresh
(f) Women wore jade–lived longer than the men
(g) Exercised in the garden

It was satisfying and a total eye-opener as far as I was concerned. From Shanghai, I headed east across the ocean to the Japanese islands of Okinawa. Many books have been written about the longevity of the people there, and we started with our meetings with Canadian professor Craig Wilcox.

Before we talk about Craig Wilcox, we will mention that from the time I landed in Guangzhou to the time I arrived back in Shanghai heading for Okinawa, I'd seen four different ethnic groups: Okinawa, Bama, Chinese Arabs, and Pakistan. That was four different countries in sixteen days, and I was well ahead of my intended itinerary thanks to the cooperation of everyone I had been with.

At that particular time, we didn't realize the importance of the fact only women wore jade and lived longer overall than the men did, even longer than the average Western woman. Moreover, there was the fact the woman up the hill had the metal bracelet on her right wrist—and as we know, metal is conductive; this gave us the first clue of the ability to keep static and imbalance from vital parts of the body until grounding takes place.

Okinawa

Okinawa used to be called Ryukyu and has been known for its longevity—a long-liver's paradise or the place of eternal youth. We refer to the study done by Professor Craig Wilcox, his brother, and Mr. Sukizu. It has had this reputation for over five hundred years. It is situated between what is now called Taiwan, Hong Kong, Japan, and Korea. It also had the reputation of being a trading nation; it has been called the Shangri-La, a marine nation with regular mixed trading between the various eastern Asian nations in the past. Obviously, with this background, there has been a creation of a new-looking race. These people do not look Japanese, and they don't look Chinese. They look a little less Asian than other Asians do, and they are smaller physically in size, but they are not actually a small race physically.

The area itself consists of over 160 islands of various sizes. It's a beautiful clean place with the different islands all having the clearest water. The people are friendly, and in the main town itself, industries are certainly up to every Western standard.

These people usually live in small groups towards the ends of the islands. There is a strong Japanese influence, as you would expect after seventy-odd years of Japanese control. The people themselves operate on the Japanese principle: timber homes and single electric lines like the Bamas. It's a bit terrifying when you look at these lines; they look like cobwebs over the entire little village, and you can't help thinking that it is strange that they are not all diseased. In fact, they appear to be the longest living and in the best condition.

I emphasize "best condition," meaning they look and act younger than of any of the nations that we are going to talk about, including the people of Bama, who *look* old. These people not only don't look old; they look thirty years younger than they are, and they act that way as well. They're fit, not overweight; they eat like the people of Bama, which is only about half of what we eat; their diet is very similar, an excess of fresh vegetables; and they have sparkling white teeth.

As stated, Okinawa was originally called the ancient kingdom of Ryukyu. They have also have a university named Ryukyu University. It had a background of strong Chinese influence, and it is only during the last seventy years, since the Japanese have taken over the area after the Second World War, that they have had a major impact on the styles and living ideas of the original Chinese background.

The Chinese appreciated this longevity in the 161-odd eastern islands that we now call Okinawa. To them, it was known as an area where you historically lived a long time. The most impressive thing about Okinawa is seeing that they still use Western medicine, particularly if they need urgent medical equipment—for example, if there is a car accident or that sort of thing. However, diseases are very rare. This longevity has been recorded as far back as many hundreds of years. You automatically believe that this has to be a genetic feature. However, if we relate the Okinawan lifestyles to the styles of the other long-living races, we will find that it's not necessarily a genetic factor. Although everybody is different and it is logical that there will be minor differences between people and families, the overall picture is turning out to be one of a number of items that they all have in common. Okinawans have intemperately Asian style. They have accurate records as to details of the birthdays of most of their population, which gives them a greater degree of authenticity regarding the long-living age.

A thing that should be mentioned here in the final analysis between the different ages and the different races is the companionship with the people in each group, which is their race. They share worries and stresses, helping individuals not to feel alone in their activities and pressures. It's almost like a socialist or tribal idea if you can relate that to our Western world.

Following the Western ideas of health, admittedly they are going to make mistakes from time to time, such as having more than two cups of coffee each day, which can be bad for you, and a week later, they tell you it's OK to have five cups of coffee each day because it is good for you or it's a good antioxidant. So things do change. Medical researchers are doing their best, and they are doing a marvellous job.

It is important to note in the Okinawans, as well as the other nations or timeless areas around the world that we have had the pleasure of examining, that when these people left their particular area and their lifestyle along with a change in their usual diet and the way they lived, they had the same problems that we do in the West, with heart disease, strokes, cancer, and so on. If they stay in their own environment and do the things that they have been doing for the past hundreds of years, these medical problems don't seem to exist to the same degree, particularly the serious diseases, such as cancer and so forth. Mammograms are unusual in that part of the world.

It is also interesting to note that people moving out of these areas seem to have the same lifespan as those living in the West! It seems that when they do this, it changes their entire living pattern, including the amount and type of exercise. Is there a link here between the changes in pattern—just like when a Western person retires from work and often the body does not quickly respond to this lifestyle change? If you were going to move from one lifestyle to another, then this would upset the body routine and its conditioned electrical balance. To be successful, you may have to keep the original lifestyle by duplicating it within the new area if you go to the Western world. In other words, this would give you the energy protection that would be needed to readjust, and likewise they would need to continue with their healthy diet and familiar exercise and routine in order to retain their good electrical balance.

Additionally, all of these races keep their body weight under control. All of these people eat plenty of *very fresh* fruit, vegetables, whole grains, and soy. In most instances, the food they have is in plentiful supply. We didn't realize at this time that we were making an important breakthrough. See the chapter on Kirlian photography and the effect on dying plants.

The Okinawa Program, Craig Wilcox's book, has more details about the different vegetables, and we will list some at the end of this discussion. As with all the different long-living races that we are talking about, Okinawan women rarely get breast cancer.

T'ai chi is usually recommended and practiced. There is another type of t'ai chi, spelt ch'uan, and this involves continuous movement. It's best that it is done with a professional teacher and, if possible, performed on grass or hard ground in bare feet outdoors. As explained earlier in the book, wearing leather or natural shoes allows a complete electrical circuit to go through the body, thereby earthing you. Having bare feet will also allow your body to be earthed. Man was not evolved to have unnatural body balance or static electricity. If you are obliged to do your exercise indoors, then do it within the principle discussed in this book and take the type of flooring into account to make sure that you are going to be grounded.

T'ai chi can start showing you physical improvement in as little as two weeks, and you should be in the swing of things in a month. If it can be used in conjunction with walking, you would be in a very strong position with your health.

T'ai chi, if done daily with your walking, tricks your body into thinking that you have completed your exercises, even if the weather makes your walking impracticable. Many good books have been written about the power of the mind (positive thinking), and any could be related to Jean and how she overcame the fear of an agonizing death. I am a student of t'ai chi, which starts by clearing your mind and removing all stress before the actual movements are involved. This way, you get maximum benefit from the exercises performed.

I walked into Okinawa University not knowing what sort of reception I was going to get. I had written to them without reply, and here I was loaded up with enough equipment to last me three months.

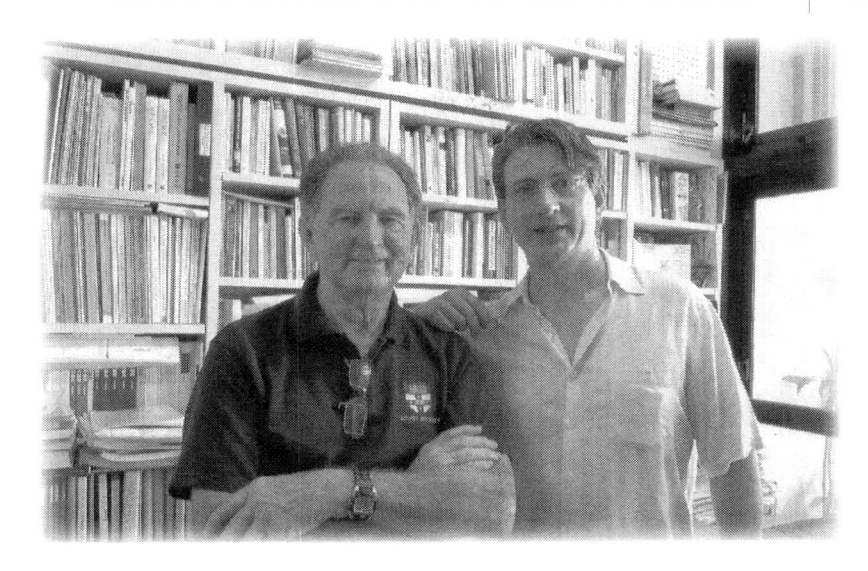

The author (left) and Craig Wilcox (right)

I knocked on the university door of Professor Craig Wilcox, co-author of the book *The Okinawa Program*. It is well worth reading and is similar to what I am trying to write. It has to do with the longevity of the Okinawan race.

I introduced myself and explained that I was trying to get comparative details between longevity of the different races around the world. I asked him how he would feel about my getting involved in such a venture and if he could help in any way. The response was as frank, understanding, and friendly as what you would expect as one researcher to another. I was delighted with his response. He explained to me that if I were to try to get anything official from any Japanese organization, it would be committee after committee. As I had spent a year in Japan myself, I knew just what he meant. He did say that there was a way of doing this, as in Australia we say "There are no flies on this guy; he is a man of action." He said the way he would do it (saying, "I don't recommend anything, of course"), and he then gave me the name of a photographer who spoke the languages of the area.

Thi fellow was on the ball, and he turned out to be surprising to look at, a little bit like what we would consider a hippy. He had a sharp brain and great photographic skills, as this was his business, and he had been involved in research before in other areas. He was exactly what I was looking for. His name was Tamio Otia. Tamio had a friend who knew where these old people were as well as the easiest way to find them.

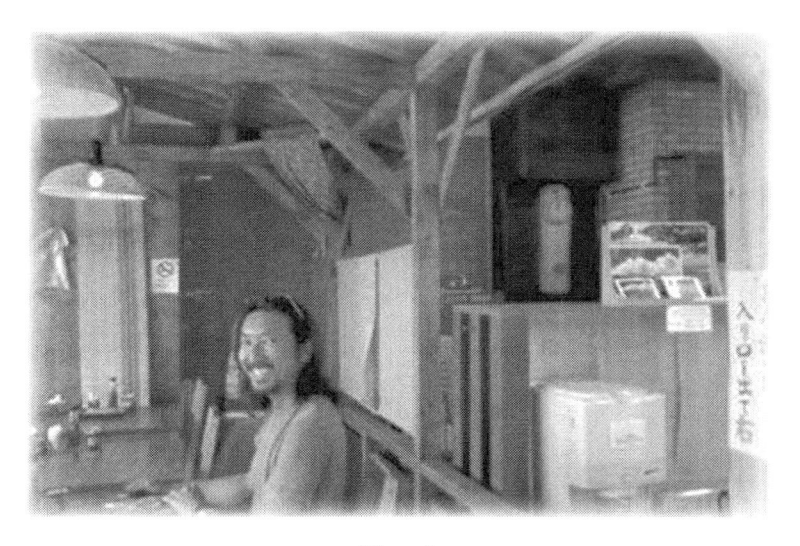

Tamio

Together the three of us (Tamio spoke perfect English) went to a village called Ogimi. Together we went to the first shopkeeper in this village, asking for a few directions. He got excited and wanted to be tested himself, and I certainly obliged. He was eighty-nine years old then, and he recorded five volts. The temperature was only eighty degrees, and the humidity was 69 per cent.

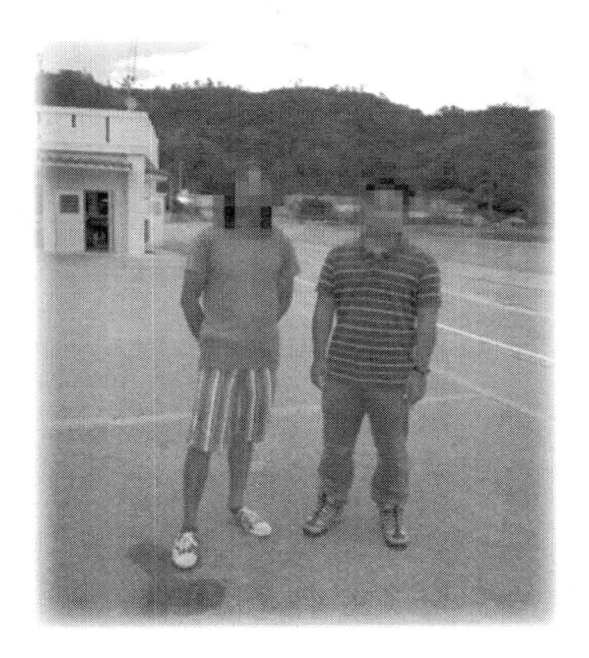

Our guides

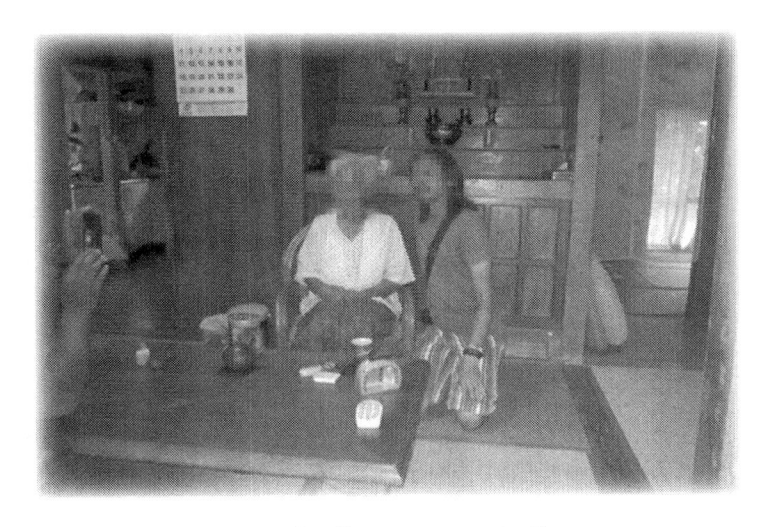

Note the flooring–static free

As a shopkeeper, he was surrounded by refrigeration and electrical gear but with surprisingly very little saleable stock on his shelves. I then had the pleasure of measuring the electrical content of Sao. She was ninety-six years old and was super fit. She walked three kilometres a day, every day, to one of her two farms, collecting wild herbs at one and growing potatoes at the other.

Okinawa has a register of births and the names and ages all registered accurately. She had a sugar cane section on her farm, she didn't eat fish, and she ate small volumes of meat and many herbs. A lively person!

Her house was timber. She was barefoot all the time in the home, and she ate grains and vegetables.

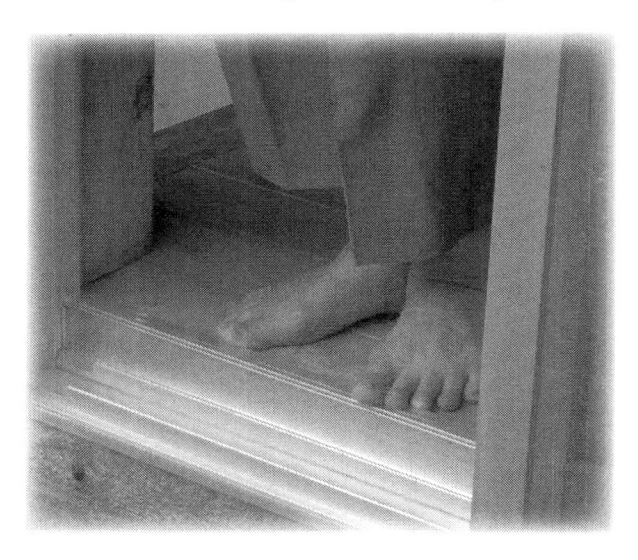

Always barefoot

Again, the house had timber floors, and she sat on the floor Japanese style. There was a fan in the room, and the home was spotless, clean, and airy. It was a nice small home with about two bedrooms, and most anybody from any Western country would be proud to live there. She had never been sick or admitted to hospital and her teeth were brilliantly white, as were those of all the people that we met in this particular town. An interesting note about this woman was that the only time she went to hospital, she was treated for poisoning from snakebite. The snake was a habu. Apparently, recently a snake bit her again, and indifferently believing it was a habu, she decided not to go to the hospital due to her physical condition. She felt fine, and there was no bad reaction at all. This is a big statement when we come to our conclusions as to the storage of energy. Interestingly, all persons in the room registered zero—no static—and everybody was shoeless in the house. This allows the body's millions of negative and positive ions to be in balance and earth you.

The next person's reading came up as one volt. She lived in a similar timber house, and she was ninety-three years old. She didn't look as young as Abu but was very pretty. Again, these people were at the bottom of a hill (this is a feature of good feng shui), near the water, with trees or a garden around, which is almost the Chinese influence, although these people, as I said, do not have the same appearances as the Chinese. This house seemed to be strongly Japanese in style, with conductive Tatami flooring over timber—personal grounding materials. The influence seemed to be more Chinese, and that applied to all the people we met there.

They had a product called *chomeigusa*; a long life grass. In addition to this, there are a number of vegetables, a range of about ten that they say are responsible for their longevity and lack of ageing. They all ate boiled pork; and they all have fish, except for one woman who didn't eat fish at all; and they had small portions of beef, goat, duck, and the vegetables in season. They only ate what they grew. They have an interesting terminology: *have haohibua*, which means half-full or half-empty. They never ate enough to be satisfied, and this is becoming a characteristic, just as it is for the people in Bama. The veggies are from terraced hillsides that are as they were hundreds of years ago, upon which they collect wild herbs daily. They sell a lot to the local restaurant, where people enjoy flavours that are most acceptable, and they have various seasons for the different vegetables and herbs. They ate more potatoes here than rice because there is not enough room to grow rice. The potato is called *beni-imo*, and it is red on both the outside and the inside.

There is no evidence of cancer in the village. The old people sell their herbs to the café, as mentioned, and they are a local specialty. A drink called ukon tea is popular there, and it's great for the liver.

Around the outside of the bay is the main power line, the thickest I have ever seen. It must have been eight inches in diameter or more, and it had a band around it, suggesting that the Japanese know what they are doing with electricity better than we do. The Japanese are amongst the world's longest-living people. I could only think that with the town in a cobweb of local power lines and a single line coming to the house itself, it was like looking at Bama again. There is always a distance between the council line to the house; it's just a single line. Having power cables too close to you causes your body's electrical balance to be in turmoil because it is unnatural. In nature, you will often see that a tree planted beneath power lines will actually grow around the electricity source—it is nature's way of protecting itself. We also need to protect ourselves from these man-made sources.

A café owner named Katsu was happy and very friendly. His mum was ninety-four years old and had a reading of zero. She was sprightly and mobile, looking twenty years younger than her age.

I reiterate again that the people we have discussed have their own vegetable gardens, with the exception of one, who had a flower garden and again were very good-looking women for their age.

The next woman had two farms and an afternoon job. She planted potatoes and was extremely fit, and so it went on ... they all had bare feet in the house. All were highly active, and all looked years younger than their actual age. There was no comparison between how they looked and the Bama people, who *looked* one hundred. When these people are one hundred, they will look sixty-five to seventy. The big punch line is that there is no sickness in the village. It starts to become obvious that if you don't get sick, you don't age, and if you don't age, you live a long time.

Momentarily going back to Bama, its location is in the Guangxi province–special reference here to Professor Craig Wilcox for supplying the Tamio Otto connection. The man was highly intelligent and helpful in every way, seeking information at every opportunity. I was proud to have him sign my report, and I would recommend him to anyone who wants such a venture.

We are starting to appreciate that we need routine exercise, where we do it repeatedly and it then becomes automatic. When working, we can also be exercising by tilling the earth, walking, or what have you. If you are in good condition and you perform the same routines daily, then this constant routine becomes practice and will not seem like work, just an everyday health regime. In other words, your work becomes your exercise, and with the right conditioning, it's not difficult. I guess it's like a bricklayer doing the same thing repeatedly. He becomes fit in the particular job, as little loss of energy is involved because it is repetitively automatic. The next extension of that is that if you have exercised and you're not exhausted, the energy you created by the exercise, which in this case would be working in the fields, is an accumulation of energy reserves that make you immune to many things, including things such as snakebites or disease.

The Okinawa's aren't fools either; they are backed by a very good hospital in the main town. One of the women mentioned that she had to have a couple of stainless bolts put in her knees. She then headed back to the fields.

BEATING CANCER WITH THE HELP OF EINSTEIN | 69

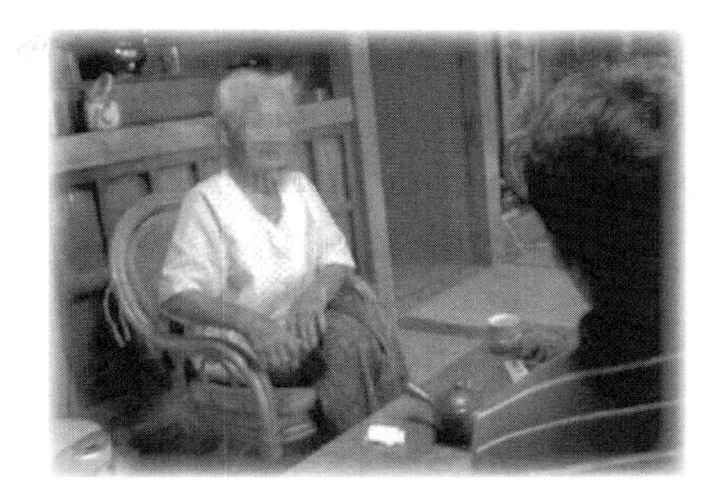

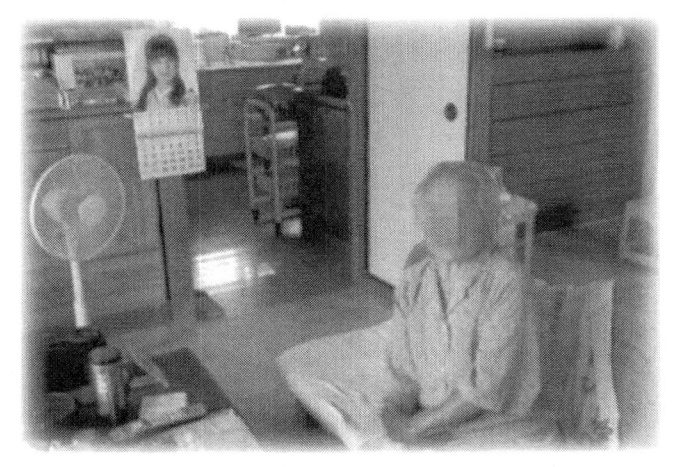

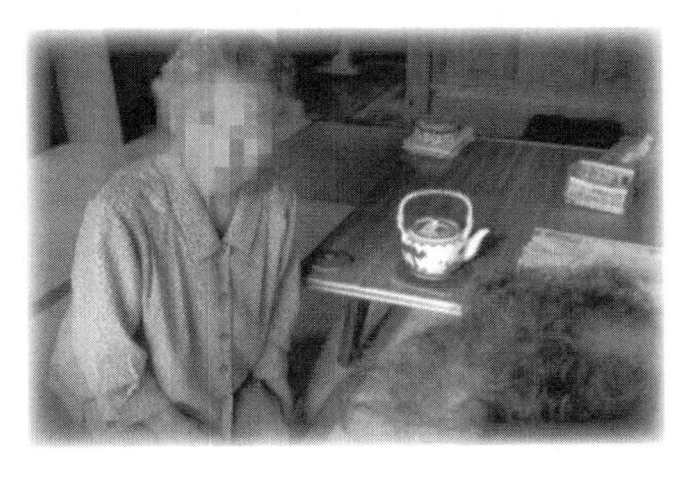

These people are prepared to work with the two different worlds, the Asian world, with its historically proven solution to disease and living a long life, and the Western medical world, where specialised medical help is required, and they are willing to use both systems if necessary. The stainless pins were needed due to heavy lifting. In addition to the physical exercise of the working people of this town, they remain conscious of the historic features and the physical exercises, such as t'ai chi, as well as traditional folk dancing and an energetic war dance using five-foot sticks in unison as a team–aggressive and violent–obviously from their history of frightening off their enemies. The sticks were depicting spears, and males apparently did the dance.

The older generation prefers to live on their land, whilst the younger generations want to be in the town, where more money can be earned, and this exposes them to health problems of the Western world. They have very strong family ties, and the family usually visits on the weekends. Families are large due to the age factor. You can find great-grandfathers and much of the extended family in the house on the weekends! As in Bama, when the younger people leave the town and go chase money, they become susceptible to the diseases of the Western world, which gives us a strong indication that locality is a big factor too. The actual location of these villages is always away from the big cities and usually a short distance from a small town. A local store could not economically survive–one store sold only some refrigerated products. The refrigerator was more like a household one, unlike the ones we have in our stores.

We found no trouble finding these people of longevity; there was no shortage of them. Again we refer you to the research done by Professor Craig Wilcox in his book titled *The Okinawa Program*. They are all sprightly, and it was obvious that those who had not reached one hundred yet were not going to have much trouble getting there, based just on their attitudes and their liveliness for their age.

One woman was greatly interested in what we were doing, but the equipment we were using ran out of batteries and we had to go try to find some sort of shop that sold anything at all–they were so self-reliant. We eventually found batteries, and on the way back, we found the same woman in the street, having been to the hills to collect vegetables and herbs. She was delighted to see us again, and we stopped on the side of the road and asked if it would be OK to take a static reading. We were surprised at her outfit. At her home, she looked like a perfectly balanced person physically, but with all the clothes she was wearing and being covered with an apron, she looked unhealthily overweight. We couldn't understand the reason for all the clothes, as the temperature was in the high eighties, and this was obviously her working gear. The hat was of great interest to us; it was made of double-sided cotton and padded.

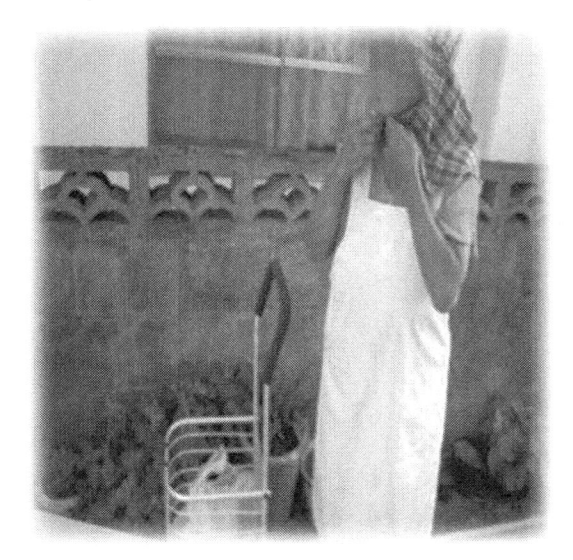

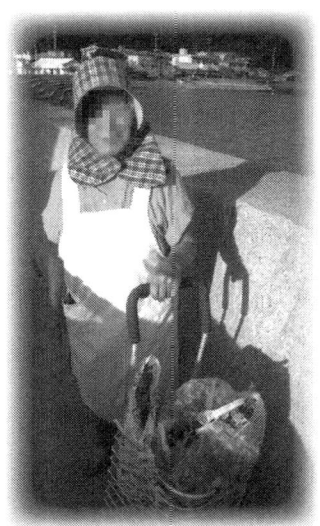

Ancient local radiation prevention outside the home?

Her reading came up as expected, just like the others in the village. I should have asked her at the time why she was wearing those garments, especially when she had been working, but I realized that it was probably to protect her against snakebite. This, of course, may not be correct.

Having convinced ourselves that we had the right readings and the right information that we needed, we headed back towards the main city with Tamio. I thanked him for his time and his knowledge and said goodbye.

The maximum static reading was 5 volts by the shopkeeper—the remainder were similar to Bama readings—you could classify the centenarians in the area static free. The temperature was 31 centigrade humity 68 per cent.

Shanghai to Urumqi, Hetian, Yutian, Layisu

I sat in the hotel room, back alone because of the language difficulties, and tried to analyse the shock of finding that these two ethnic groups had the same personal electrical comparisons–close to identical. This was becoming a justification of the possibility of some sort of breakthrough with my wife and mother.

I had two possibilities of two groups left, not too far from where I was. I decided upon these groups because they were well known for their longevity. One was located in the town of Layisu, via Urumqi Hetian, which required me to go towards the top and around the outside of the western side of China, making many stops to get to this isolated spot. I had no idea what to expect when I got there after starting from Shanghai.

The other alternative was to fly from Shanghai to Islamabad, to the volatile area and the only place where I knew that I could get weapons–so far, I had never found it necessary to carry any weapons, even travelling alone. But I knew where I could buy weapons at the entrance of the Khyber Pass. I knew what they would cost, and I had the cash with me. It took me back to the days when Jean and I were last there, where you could actually buy any weapon on the northern side of the pass that you needed, including M14 and M16 rifles, pistols, and even rocket launchers if you needed them. It was a bit like the last time when we were in Guam, where after a ten-day notice, you could load your boat with weapons to defend yourself against the pirates, necessary if you were travelling west from Guam.

The downside of this Pakistan area was that I would still be travelling alone. It was a magical place because you could stand outside the gun shop and watch the trucks accumulate after they had received their guards to guide them down Khyber Pass. You could look up and see the Pakistan guard post on the hill above the gun purchasing area, which was only a few hundred yards away, and I will never forget the sight of a camel train of a dozen camels heading in a south-westerly direction, fully loaded and on trails that possibly have never been marked. Although it was a magical scene, as I stood there, I thought of the turmoil in Pakistan. I would have to get from this area to Hyderabad because I would then jump off to the mountainous Hunza scene.

But I did need a third verification from an ethnic group that they all had this one feature in common: constant personal grounding. From that, we can form the basis of a possible cure or at least an extension of life.

Because of the safety of China and the fact that I was appreciating the value of the information that I was collecting and recording, I elected to go and find this ethnic group on the China-Vietnam border. Not knowing what to expect, I headed for Shanghai as a starting point.

Islamabad, Pakistan

I parked myself in the hotel for the night and organized my next trip. We had two choices: to try to get to Islamabad in Pakistan and then to the Khyber Pass, as this was the only place that I knew of where I could buy weapons. It is a highly volatile religious area as mentioned earlier, and everyone carries a gun.

I'd need this equipment, and I would need guards that could speak English. In my opinion, the guards I had had in the past in that area were not robust or dedicated persons and wouldn't be tough enough should there be a showdown. The equipment they were using was extremely dated, and they did not ask for much money for remuneration.

From there, we could go forward, to the area of the Hunzas, in the Hunza Valley, if I could get the right guards.

As I sat in the hotel that night, the information that I had made me realize that I was on the verge of actually achieving a breakthrough as far as the human viewpoint is concerned in the prevention of disease. I became conscious all of a sudden of the value of my own research that I had carried out.

I had another option, of course, and that was to head for Layisu, within the Chinese government protection and on the border with Vietnam. It was a difficult place to get to at any time, but I felt that this would be a much safer way to travel.

Hotan, or Hetan, as it can be known

The information–the readings from the machine of the centenarian's electrical balance that I had already gathered–was consistent, with only slight variations between the different locations but all coming down to the same end results. I really felt the importance of this information but thought that I should firstly verify and check these consistencies to avoid mistakes with even more examples. The trek was a long one, with no English expected along the way.

I headed off the following morning, and eventually, after many flights and bus trips, I got to the town of Hotan. This was an absolute revelation. I felt lost as soon as I got into the town, as there was no English spoken anywhere and no Westerners at all. I got into the hotel making sign language to try to get a room, which I eventually got. I had no idea what I was paying for the accommodation; I just held out the notes in my hand, and they took what was necessary. It was embarrassing on their part as well as for me. I then made more enquiries about the town and found that there was an international hotel around the corner. I booked a room there instead, and when asking if anyone spoke English, I found a beautiful young Chinese woman who could speak quite acceptable English.

Hotan—modern town, old ideas

She ran the restaurant part of the hotel. The food was excellent, of course, and the service was good because I could make myself understood and I could get information. By coincidence, she said she had the next day off and could take me to these old people, and she said the town of Hotan was full of old people, centenarians. However, while I was talking to her, unexpectedly a fit young fellow, a local named Jilil, said he would be happy to take me. His English was nine out of ten. He had a vehicle, and I explained that I was prepared to pay for his time. He said that would be all right, and off we went to meet the Layisu, a tribe some distance away from Hotan. Hotan itself turned out to be a very interesting place; the people were not Chinese, although there was a Chinese influence there.

There had been political or racial trouble in the past, and a force of riot police in their full riot gear and carrying big shields came marching through the town to let people know that the town was policed and disciplined. The town was very calm, nothing like Bama. These people were much like the Turks in appearance, and the guide himself pointed this out. We could have actually been in Turkey, as they had the same colour of skin and mannerisms. They were a wiry- looking breed and friendly, but all of a sudden, I realized that there were as many shops selling jade as we would find selling women's clothes in our own country. It was a surprise to realise that we were in a jade hub or marketplace. The area was famous for the black and white jade. There are various types of jade, and all have different healing powers, depending upon the minerals they contain.

The town was spaciously set out. Some of the roads were a good forty yards wide. There were not a lot of cars in the area, although there were some. There were wood carriers selling their timber, pulling their carts around. The bakery (see photographs) will give an idea of the lifestyle of the people.

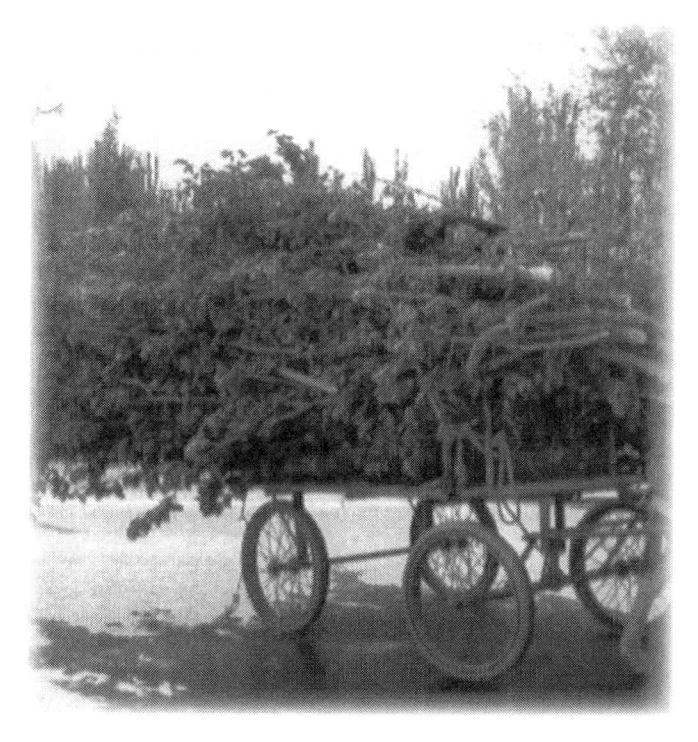

Wood carriers

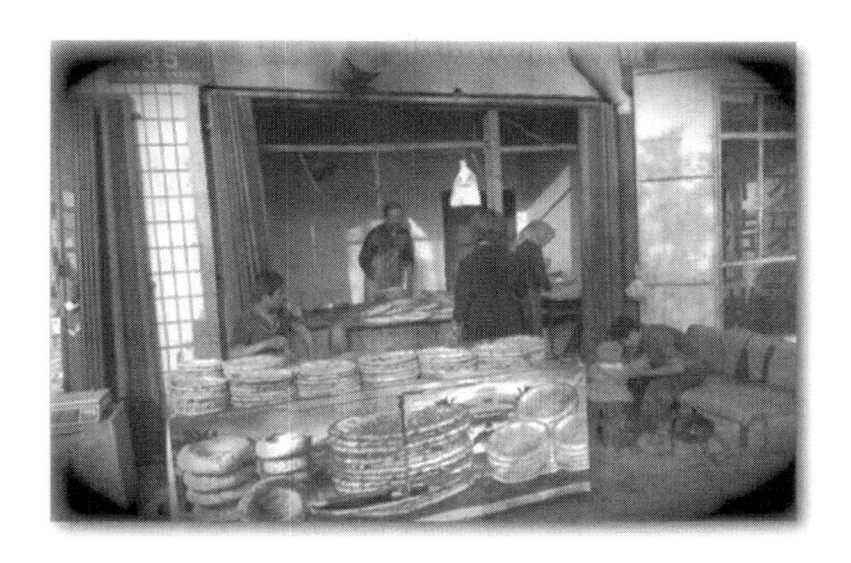

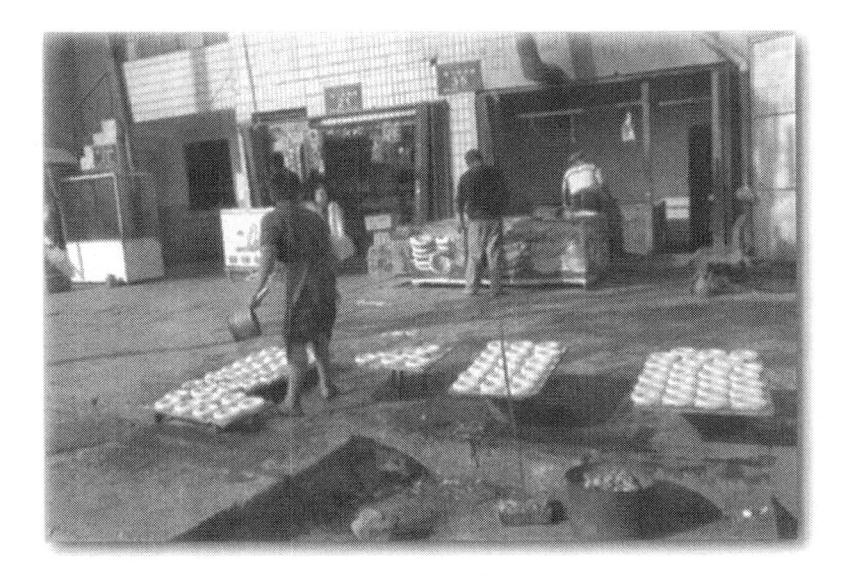

Street bakery

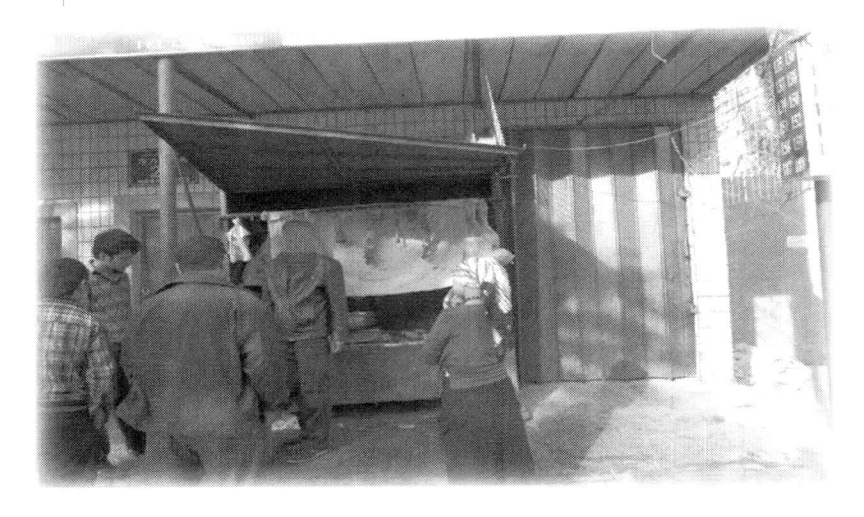

Meat market

They were cooking their pancake-type bread in the street, but there were not a lot of people in the streets. It was a shock to find an ethnic group as part of China. I agreed to meet Jilil at the Westlake's international hotel the next morning to go see the old people. I hadn't had breakfast, so I invited him to have breakfast with me at the hotel. He responded by thanking me and pointed out that he didn't eat that type of food. He then invited me to have breakfast with him in his normal restaurant. He was actually building a restaurant himself down the road, but he had that day off. We went to his restaurant, and I found it most interesting. We sat in bench-type seats as one might do in the army. The food was in a large bowl with soup-type ingredients, and it took two hands to lift the bowl to your mouth. The taste was outstanding. I cannot describe the pleasure it gave me, and I thoroughly enjoyed it. What was particularly interesting was that after we had eaten and gone to his car, I felt physically elated. I was feeling like an athlete, full of energy and super fit, and I had the sensation of wanting to do a run or compete in a sport. I remembered feeling like this when I was young! I also remembered thinking that if one could feel like this after eating, there was some money to be made here, especially if you could put it in a can. I said this to Jilil, and he laughed. I don't know what I actually ate or drank. I think it was a mutton type broth—a most enjoyable experience.

We left in Jilil's smart vehicle after I assured him that I had no political interest in his town, as it was a very unusual situation for a Western person to be in this part of the world. He was satisfied, so off we went. It was like a drive through the desert. It was dusty, and there was nothing to see as we drove down a beautifully wide two-lane road, unusual because it was an outback road and not a city one, and this would be uncharacteristic even in the Western world. The road seemed to go nowhere, and the drive seemed to take a long time.

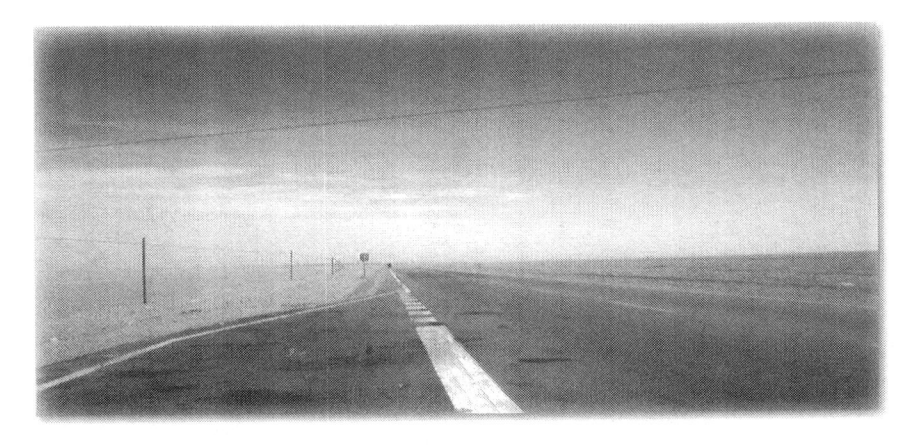

Road to nowhere

We didn't pass any other vehicles or persons in either direction. The useless ground on the right side of the road was scrubby and grassless, just like you would find in outback Australia. The left-hand side of the road followed the edge of a desert that looked like it contained Sahara-type sand hills.

We eventually came to the town. We could see it coming due to the rows of poplars, which you find growing where there is shallow water below the ground– it let us know that there could be vegetation found in that particular area. On arriving in the town itself, I saw that the houses were mud-type dwellings. There were very few people around. We went first to the council chambers; the floor was dirt in the compound area.

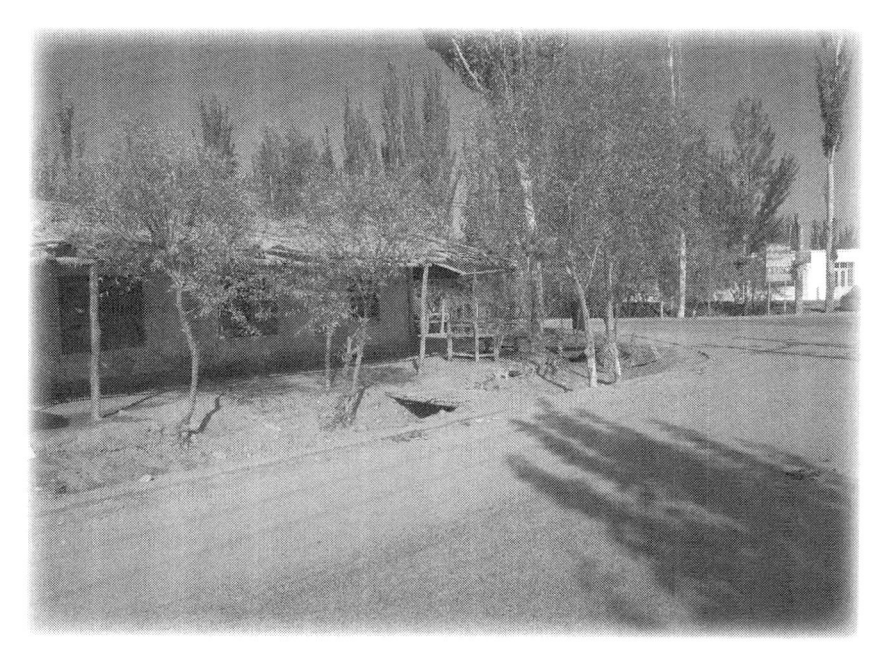

Local house

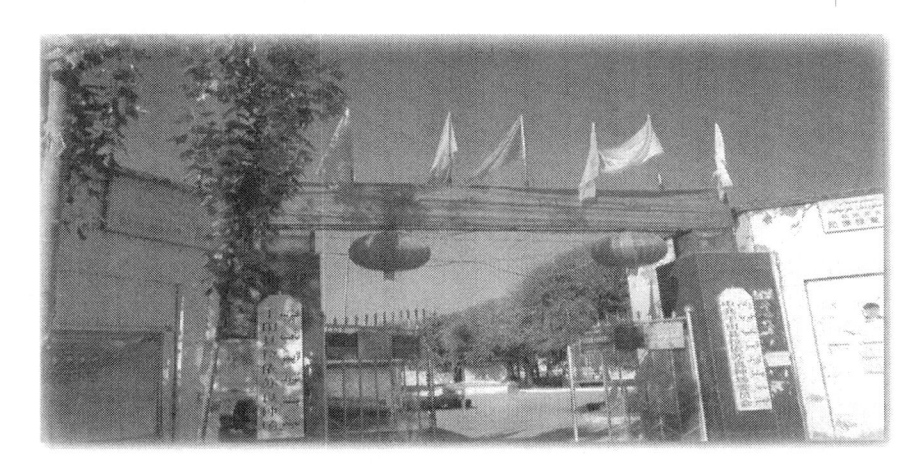

The council chambers

There were some flags up, but the scarcity of people was quite surprising. We drove around for a while and eventually came across their paddocks of vegetables, or herbs, as they call them. It was the first time I had ever seen a mini tractor in any of the old people's areas. There was a river nearby, and I realized quickly that when knocking on the door of these little compounds of about a half acre or more, the subterranean water was almost at ground level—thus when you dug a hole, you could almost see the water, which was only about one foot under the ground (see photo). Most of the town was actually built on a water table, thus the intensive growth of poplars, which gave them the wood for their fires.

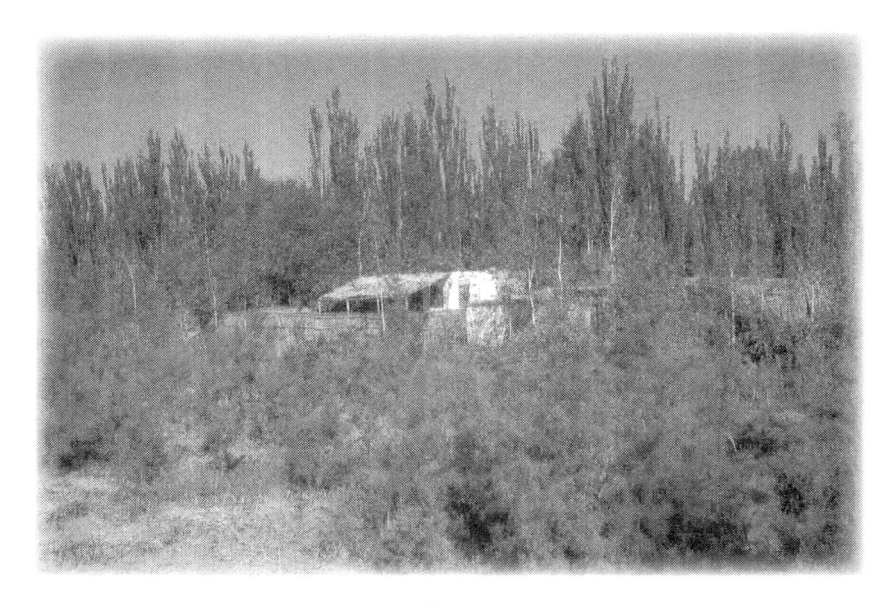

Poplar trees

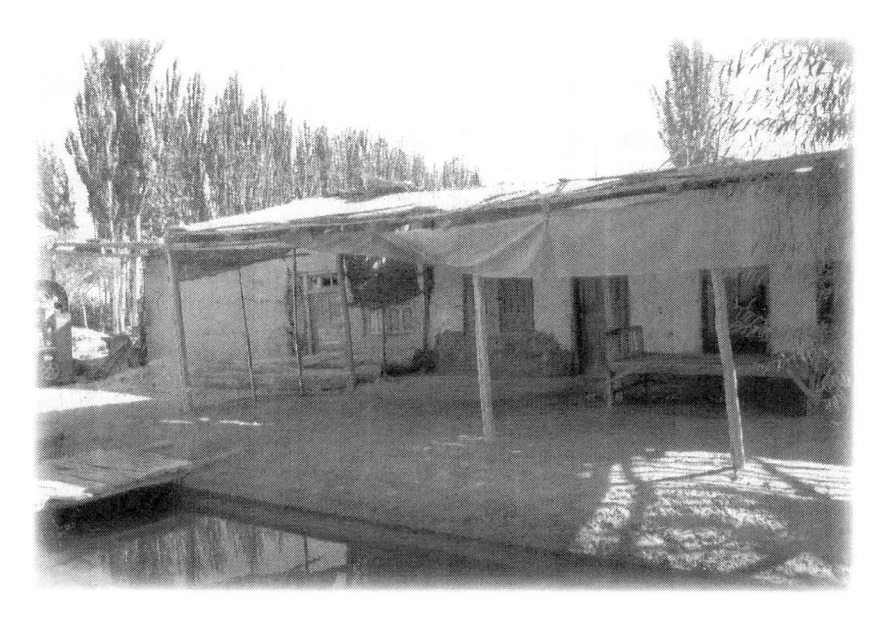

Homes with water in front

Many of them had a single electrical cable going to their homes. The sleeping beds were typically about a foot or more above the floor, which usually consisted of river stones cemented together. It made walking a bit difficult for a person like myself, who was used to walking on a flat area. We met two people who were of great interest. One was 103 and named Matohti; he still worked on the farm every day. He was very sprightly. I walked up the road with him, and he out walked me without even trying, as this was his natural walk.

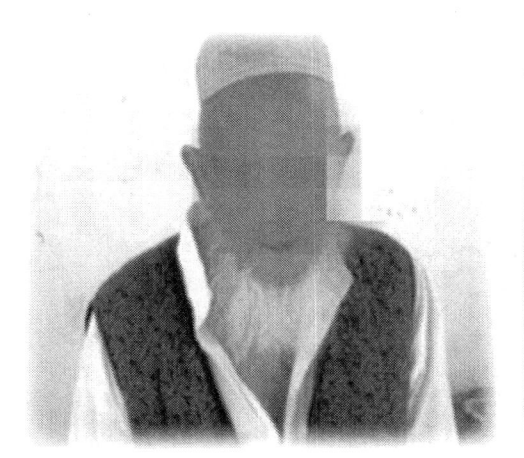

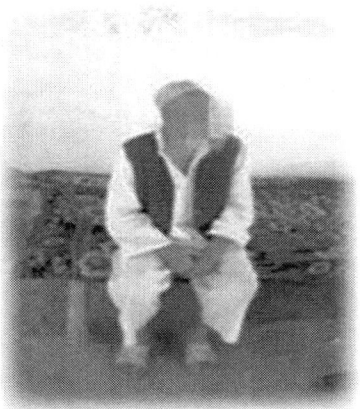

The other was 108 and named Matturzi; he had just retired. Thick dust was everywhere. The principal food at that particular time seemed to be corn–just masses of corn everywhere! The photographs of these two interesting people are included. We came across other long-livers in the town, and they just looked like the people in Hotan.

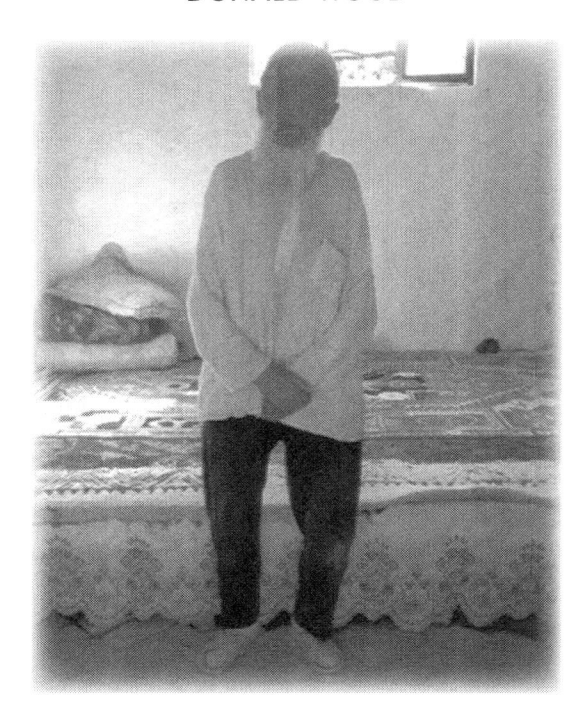

The consistently low readings were what you would expect from someone in natural electrical balance. They were disease-free, the same as all these old people. Their work was their exercise, and the food was obviously a good balance of veggies and sheep.

We met other younger people there, and again, as I mentioned, they looked like the people in Hotan. There was no Chinese influence there at all. They all wore religious cap, being Muslim, I think. They were unshaven, as we had found in other Chinese areas. You could imagine that they would look much younger had they been shaven. All were alert. We were getting the same electronic results as we had from the previous old people.

I felt that the information that I now had was conclusive in that static electricity does not exist in these particular areas. Civilization has not caught up with them, and as a result, we have a disease-free location.

We came back to Hotan the same way we left, down this long straight road, and I said goodbye to Jilil. He asked if I wanted to see more of the local people–these oldies. I said I had the information that I needed. It was conclusive–three different areas with the same readings and similar results. Compared with the Western world this is actually a mind-blowing example of consistency. If you don't get diseases, you don't grow old to the same extent. Once you get disease, it affects the ageing process.

Jilil confirmed that the area was, as far as he knew, cancer-free. I thanked Jilil for his time, wished him all the best with his restaurant, and said that I hoped one day we would meet again. He was a likeable and physically healthy young fellow.

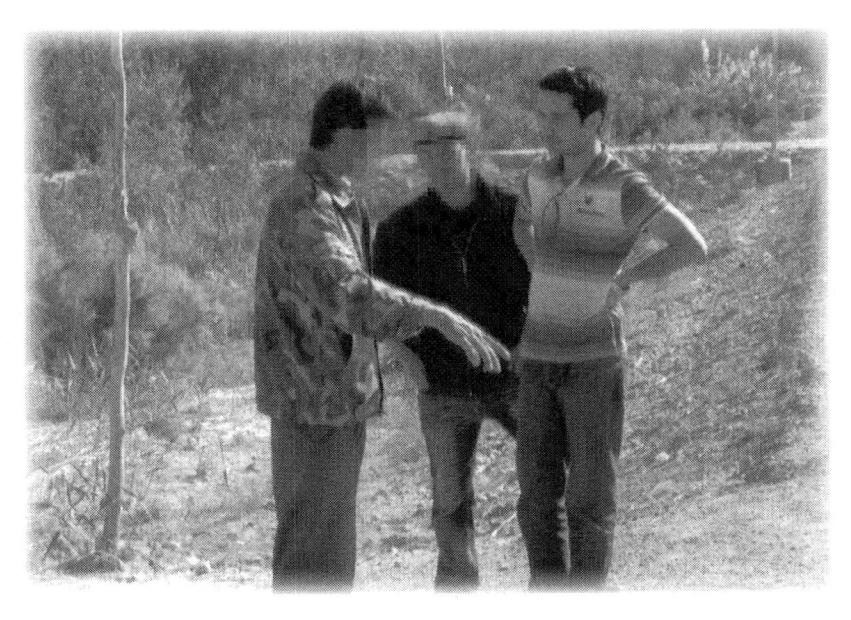

Locals with guide Jilil (blue shirt)

Hunzas from the mountainous valley in the Gilgit-Balistan region of Pakistan are very well documented, probably the most documented and closely studied of the ancients of the longevity people, but they are not the longest livers. These exist north of Bama, where the oldest person in the world, according to the records available to us, was 124, a male; the longest living female, at 118, also lived in the area.

The Hunza's are physically more like the Okinawan's in their ability to play highly competitive sports. When they look about seventy years old, they are actually over one hundred.

The Layisu and Hunza have masses of poplar trees around them, which satisfies a lot of their timber needs. A lot of them use kerosene lamps. In Hunza, power is available, but they don't want to have interference from the Pakistani government. They had an option of the government treating their wine crop with insecticides, but they refused to have any chemicals near their town at all, and they developed their own nontoxic method of protecting their crops from bugs in the summertime.

When asked what makes the people live for so long, the past local Hunza mayor, Mir (their leader), said it was the water. They were getting massive amounts of beautiful water full of minerals from the Himalayas, and of course that would have a great bearing, but no one had ever measured the amount of static electricity in their bodies. If he had said that it was because they were not involved in the Western world and therefore had no static, he would have been 100 per cent correct.

It should be noted that the people in all these areas generally use their own effluent to fertilize the ground, and this has been done repeatedly for many hundreds of years. They don't use chemicals. The bacterium is natural to them, and as they are farming and living together, that bacterium has become common and acceptable to their bodies. Because of their isolation, no foreign bacterium is introduced. Foreign bacteria would cause illness because it wouldn't balance favourably within their own bodies. Without disease, there is a longer lifespan, but those youngsters who leave to chase money in the big cities don't have any resistance to the Western world's diseases, whereas their parents who stay at home don't have to contend with those diseases because that challenging bacteria does not generally exist.

Another thing all areas had in common was that most of the cooking was still done with timber offcuts. This is not easy to find, and usually there are wood collectors that go around the streets selling their wares, namely the timber. Because of supply and demand, it is not cheap, so naturally they don't do the volume of cooking. They don't cook the goodness out of the product. They work on the principal that lightly cooked or not cooked at all is better for you, and they are right.

Fate and luck had brought me to make a wrong decision—everything was a win. It took a lot less time than expected due to the cooperation I received. For those people whom I haven't thanked, please accept this as my thanks.

When I came back, I thought about what to do with the information we'd obtained, and this is where things got interesting. We didn't want to find ourselves in a situation where we have this information and cannot use it to stop the diseases in the Western world. We now have the clues. A parallel group of features exists that applies to all of the above ethnic groups.

- Is it genetic? No. They experience the same diseases we do once they move to the Western world.
- Is it lack of static? Yes. There is no static, as their bodies are in balance.
- Is it location? Definitely. The old people are often found in small groups. As previously mentioned, everything surrounding them is familiar and natural to them—even bacteria.
- Is it food? Yes. The food is super fresh and still living.
- What about stress? Their lifestyle is stress-free.

There could also be a missing link—something we just don't understand at this time, related to location maybe!

But how are we going to use this information? How does Jean's miracle fit into the above? It is all about eating fresh food, exercising, maintaining a good electrical body balance, living stress-free, and avoiding static.

It's no good unless we can apply it to both our Eastern and Western worlds—but we can. We can show why most serious Western medicines have and will continue to fail, as well as the options. This is a big statement, a controversial one as well, but it offers alternative solutions to stopping diseases.

Obviously, we need to see if we can get Westerners to produce the same static results as the centenarians.

Life is like riding a bicycle. To keep your balance, you must keep moving.
– Albert Einstein.

CHAPTER 7

Western and Ancient Worlds

ALL AREAS IN this big world vary, each having their ways and benefits, and I feel that we could all work together and help one another. In our Western world, we have the medical know-how, for instance, to help people who have suffered a stroke, whereas in other part of the world, people could still be dying from that very thing. We could incorporate some of the ideas of the centenarians into our Western ways and even use our techniques to help them. Who knows—their 100 years might just stretch out to 130 or 140! So we can help each other here by not closing our minds to the overall picture.

The fact of the matter is that we are in the Western world, and we have to live with that. The solution is to understand why we are dying and be able to use the great benefits of this Western world. Once we know why we are dying, then we can at least put, as I mentioned herein, our defences into action or show people how to do it. We can't rely on the government or big business to do it; we need to do this at a personal level.

I feel people are dying now needlessly. The medical profession does not consider grounding or static-related problems when diagnosing patients. Until they stand up and take these things into consideration, people will die! People should or could have their electrical body balance checked prior to administering medication, and their living environment should be examined to see whether that is a contributing factor towards their disease. Constant grounding should be an important factor within the home and office as well. Clean air is important. Should the outside air be contaminated or come from a contaminated source, a wind vane would indicate the direction of this source. You could then open another window where the wind source comes from a cleaner environment and add clean air to your home. There is no industry around the area where the centenarians live, and they make sure that their homes are aerated all the time.

It is very important that we keep in mind that we shouldn't adopt the Western world's attitude of "wait until you get a disease and then cure it". The attitude should be to stop getting those diseases in the first place so we don't have to try to cure them, which we had to do with my loving wife, Jean. We should examine our daily actions; this is very important to ensure that our physical actions are repetitive, and if you find that they are not long-term repetitive, find a way of making them so.

Even when you walk to work or walk to the bus, you are exercising, and your body will grow to expect it. If your medical practitioner suggests that you have a weakness in some part of your body but you currently have no disease, work on fixing that weakness. If you are pregnant, don't allow your baby to inherit your health problems. Take precautions to protect the area where your little one is housed (your "baby bump"). Wear a fabric shield, covering the area so you don't increase the risk of adding possible health problems or weaknesses to his or her DNA. It will save you money in the long run by way of medical expenses. It might save you thousands or even a cherished life.

If you must have air conditioning, make sure that you find other means of ventilation and energy, take a walk, move your feet up and down, and avail yourself of good clean air, to build up your energy reserves so that you have something to try to balance the ions that you are losing if you are in an unhealthy area. Perhaps open the doors and/or go for a quick walk or have a few stretches, anything that increases your activity level.

A gentle breeze of good air blowing through an area is essential, but of course, differences vary as to what is a reasonable amount of circulation. Take it up with the people who are running these places, as it gets those ions working, and the body balances back into its original state, as it was designed to be. As far as possible in hospitals and those locations, keep in mind that you should be trying to quickly get back to your normal routine. This is important; when you have conditioned your body to a regular routine, the sooner you get back to it, the better it is for your body. Your body is waiting for it–as any athlete would know.

If you are retiring and are going to leave that routine that you have had and feel you are in pretty good shape, then try to duplicate a similar exercise. Try to keep active. Make sure that the routine that you have had in the past or a similar routine that your body is expecting is still going to be there. Gradually wean your body from one exercise type to another. I feel that walking is the best idea because you don't have to think about it. We should point out that by exercising you are building up your energy levels, which helps you fight disease and static. You may have had to run for a bus every morning, and you used to find it rather easy. Then do exactly the same thing: don't go for a walk; go for a run.

The idea is to keep the routine going, the same as the oldies around the world are doing. They have their heads in the dirt a lot of the time–get down there and do a bit of gardening as a routine. It is all about routine. Your body is expecting it. The body was designed to do just that.

Eat good foods and keep your eye on your weight. If Jean neared the sixty kilos, she would regulate her food intake. Make sure you have breakfast as often as possible, including soft materials, such as porridge. For her breakfast, Jean always had fruit. It did not have to be fresh fruit; it could have come out of a container. She drank lots of tea. She made sure that she kept herself hydrated all the time. She would have a glass or two of wine at night, but I never saw her intoxicated.

If you play golf or bowl and find you are totally exhausted at the end of the game, you are not in condition. Work on that. Include more walking or running exercises. Concentrate on earthing by having the correct footwear so your body is constantly in contact with the ground when you are walking.

The current shoes in the marketplace isolate you and require you to do a lot of work. Whereas if your shoes were properly grounded and made of leather rather than synthetic, you would have better body balance and would accumulate more energy within your body, which would allow you to exercise more and with less effort. You will notice that t'ai chi people are always barefooted. They are grounded all the time, accumulating energy.

Don't be averse to creating other exercises, particularly stretching exercises, as well as other sports. If you are totally exhausted at the end of these particular sports that you have played, then you must build up your condition to handle those sports, just as you would build it up to handle walking or jogging. You are not looking for complete exhaustion at the end, for that is not good for you. The sporting coaches' terminology of "No pain, no gain" does not apply, because when your sporting championships are over, you cannot naturally get back to the "winning" condition again. The idea is to progressively build it up so that when you finish your squash or whatever sport, you are still quite competent to have another small session. Work out a way of enjoying your exercise. Consciously think of happy things—your girlfriend or your partner and the good times you are having. Try not to worry about things. Write down your problems and how you are going to solve them and then consider carrying through with the solutions.

Analyse the clothes that you are wearing both at work and at home in relation to not creating static. The best idea as far as footwear is concerned is to take your shoes off when you walk into a house. This could be a bit more difficult to do in an office; you might talk to the boss about it. For example, wool on wool is good, but synthetics on wool are not good, and this applies to the suit or any other things you are wearing.

In your vehicle, if you can afford leather seats, this solves many problems, but it still leaves a vehicle full of static because of the tyres. We will be talking to the motor industry about that.

I am looking at ways of reducing static in the bedroom—after all, as they say, you spend one-third of your life in bed. Satisfying sex can make many problems disappear by relieving the stresses of the working day.

As far as food is concerned, gradually cut your meals down. The average person is overweight. We should try to cut food down to about half of what we would normally eat. Understand diet and eat good things. This is one of the reasons Australians have some of the longest lifespans in the world.

We need to take our living techniques back to those of thousands of years ago but at the same apply the current brilliance of Western medicine to our situation as it is today. We need to get our bodies' electrical balance back in order individually, and by doing this, we will have a chance of doing what the Western world's medicos are trying to achieve.

The ancient world has it medical solutions derived from hundreds and thousands of years of trial and error. They don't know why, but many of their ways *do* work very well. Here in the Western world, we work on the principal that you *must* understand why it happens, but the ancients work on the principal that if it works, use it! The elements that could possibly do harm have been written out of their techniques through sheer trial and error. I am using the Chinese here as an example because their documentation, their written word, goes back about two and a half thousands years BC and there is a lot of information about it.

They believe in feng shui and choose to live in the right place. The negative ions that come over the hills are in effect working on balancing their bodies. Their repetitive exercise, mainly in the agricultural fields, means that their bodies are constantly accumulating energy to fight off disease.

We too are an ethnic group–a newer, different type– and we have created a monster with electricity, which we just can't handle. All ethnic groups vary in one way or another, so we don't only need one way of defeating disease–*our way*, our Western medicine way!

CHAPTER 8

Static Electricity

COMPARING STATIC ELECTRICITY to normal electricity, normal electricity is live electricity, which has a current, but static electricity does not have a current, and it is electricity that is out of balance. This phenomena is usually only found in nature in electrical storms and is chiefly created accidentally as a result of our endeavours and inventions to make our world more so-called civilized.

This static electricity–this unbalanced electricity–is an electricity that searches for grounding in order to achieve a normal balance of positive and negative. Until it finds this balance or this grounding, it can actually accumulate in strength to an excessive voltage to which the human body was never evolved to handle.

We know now that static causes the body to be imbalanced and in turn can expose the person to diseases–radio-transmitting towers do not discriminate whether it is electromagnetic radiation or static. Static leaves a person in danger of getting diseases, and the danger may be worse than expected. More research is needed urgently–independently and free of big business.

By grounding at a personal level, you can be in a position to counter-attack before disease takes hold–the old-fashioned body balance way, not the Western way of fixing the disease after it's established!

A new study in Brazil has shown that radio towers have caused seven thousand deaths in Brazil's third largest populated city. Because of tower radiation exposure, serious diseases not only in adults but also in children include breast, liver, and kidney problems. The danger area is worked out to be within one-third of a mile of the tower. This comes from *The Watcher* of June 24, 2013.

We concluded that there was a relationship between static electricity and radiation. Peter Staheli's research proved that weeping power lines were causing static electricity. These power lines were upsetting the bioelectrical life process, causing cancer and premature ageing. A more popular theory is that radiation is causing this shortening of life, disease, and death.

After Jean died, research came out showing that electrical power outlets–or power points, as we call them in Australia–give off radiation. This information was not available to us before that, and we believed that our home was a type of shield, giving us protection because of its location and how we had set the home up.

Experiments with the power points in the home showed that that Peter Staheli was correct. If we got within twenty-nine inches (and Jean would have been right on that verge when she was sleeping) from a power point, it would have an unnatural effect on that person. The following information is vitally important, and other researchers will use this information as a possible cure in the future.

If a Winky shield were placed between the power point and the instrument measuring voltages, both static and radiation, then a person would be protected. (See photograph 1, with fabric shield between instruments and power points.)

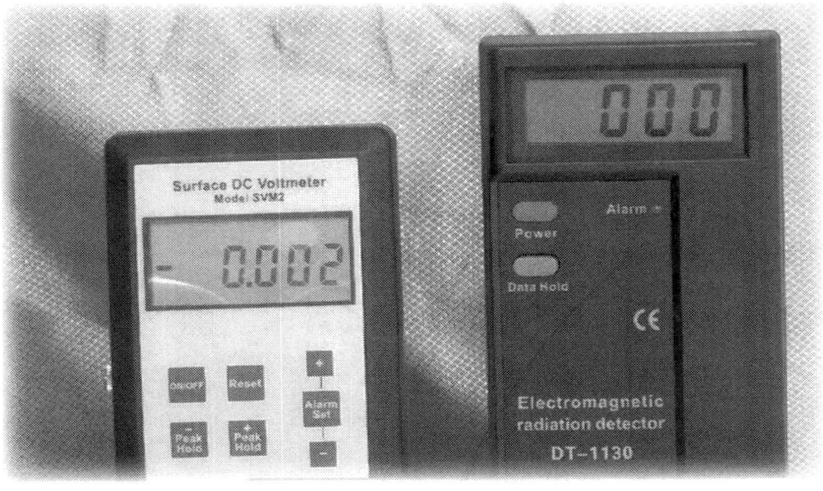

Photo 1 With fabric shield behind

The fact is, *both* were stopped. If we removed the shield (the fabric), then both items give us a result, indicating that the weeping power point is emitting both radiation and static together. (See photo 2.)

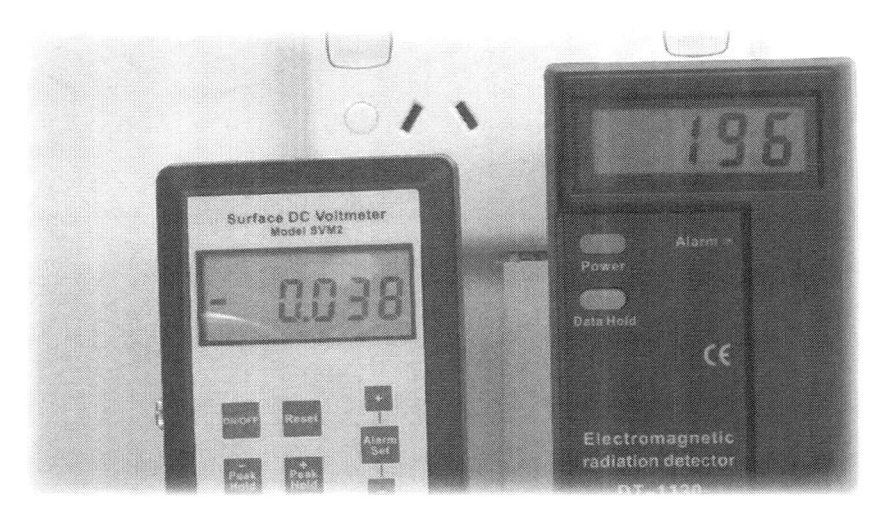

Photo 2

In photo 3, you will notice that we have had some sort of an interruption to the power strength, and it's important to note that the percentage of decrease from photo 2 to photo 3 is close to consistent, indicating that they are actually *related*. As one drops, it affects the amount the other one drops. For example, the static drops and the radiation drops proportionately until none exists, as the shield is protecting you.

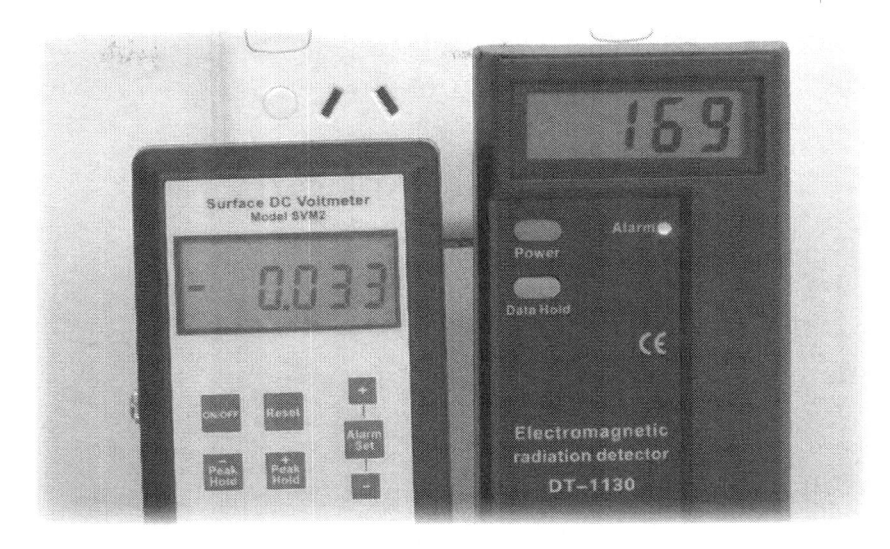

Photo 3

This indicates, of course, that if we can get rid of one of these two items, then the other will follow suit. This gives researchers the opportunity of understanding what is happening and what is necessary for them to handle to solve the problem.

Note: The drop in result may be proportional between static and at least one type of radiation, and we know how to control static. Of course, it should be noted that various factors can change this situation, valuable as it is. We would have to consider this generalizing at this time, as a complete book could have been written on the importance of this information. Should we not be talking about a power point in this instance but referring to a human body having this degree of static, and as previously mentioned there is a link between static and radiation, if you reduce the static in the body, then automatically the radiation is reduced as well. It makes one wonder if there is a link between wearing non-natural fabrics, which can cause static, and perhaps some radiation and breast cancer.

Again, we all vary to some extent—even twin brothers or twin sisters are not likely to die on the same day unless in an accident together. There are different variations in our make-up that make us a little different from even the closest family relatives. We have to find out whether those ethnic groups have one particular gene or factor that is different from ours in the Western world. Now fate has taken a hand in this report, and as fate would have it, again an opportunity came along to allow me to prove one way or another that what these people have is different from what we have in the electrically civilized world.

My family was bringing a sailing yacht from Europe to Australia and had arrived in the British Virgin Islands in good condition, but they had a need for some additional crew to take them across the notoriously rough waters between the Caribbean and the Panama Canal. I accepted their invitation to try to help them in this transit. My mind flashed back to thirty years previously, to the yachtsman who returned cured of leukaemia.

When Westerners are isolated from civilization, they are free from the effects of electricity and static, which is what we experience by being on the sea. Mostly wind generation and solar power created the power. The engine was used only for generating additional power, which was unusual because of the wind forces, which averaged just under forty knots for the transit. The power needed was only 12 volts, not 120 or 240 volts.

There would be four of us on board, and as expected, the conditions were particularly rough because of the counter current that runs back from the power of the winds hitting the seaboard of the eastern Americas. This is the reverse current to a great extent, and it made the trip very bumpy, so much so that it was quite common to have water in the cockpit. We were thrown around quite dramatically due to the turbulence of the water. Two very important things happened as a result of that: Firstly, without exception, everybody on that boat was grounded 100 per cent, as it was necessary to activate H.F. and hand emergency radios if needed; the boat had to be grounded electrically for the radios to work– grounding the four crew on the boat, taking us back personally to the grounding level of the ethnic groups, so it is not a genetic thing.

Secondly, while we occasionally had minus numbers with the ethnic groups, every reading I took of the electronics on the boat showed a minus reading as low as minus four. This is a very low reading, but questions come to my mind here in relation to Albert Einstein's sister. She was in the turbulent water areas of Davos, being bombarded, possibly not as great as we were on the boat but still to a certain extent, by good negative ions. She would have had leather shoes on in the early 1930s. Grounded as we were in bare feet, we found ourselves in the same situation.

People are often recorded laughing after storms, as personal elation is a feature of negative ions. I can say that we hardly stopped laughing from the time we got on that boat and went to sea to the time we got to the Panama Canal. It was a very happy, loving, and fun trip, and we were in a strong healing scenario but *not* an ethnic group. We have to keep our body in electrical balance just like the electronics in a car; if you let it get out of balance, it will affect the rest of car.

Ideally, we hope to make a preventative product that we will call a Winky. This product will prevent most of the static and radiation from getting to any vulnerable areas you might have. We suggest covering baby bumps and breasts using the Winky shield. There is a lot to do in getting all these inventions and principals up and running.

With information that we have gathered from these efforts, I feel that we can safely build on this. If many millions of people are going to die from diseases this year, then there is a degree of urgency to give them the same chances that Jean had.

Radio waves—the solution

As proof that this works, if you were to wave a key card (a hotel room key) in front of the lock of a door, the key card would automatically register the details and the door lock would be activated and released. However, if you were to place this particular fabric between the door lock and the card itself, you would find that it doesn't work, indicating that the electric pulses are not getting through to the door; in the same way, the electronic pulses cannot get through or into your body.

Particular metals can cause skin irritations. In every instance when this is happening and you don't feel well, you should remove the metal item. The only metal that appears to have nil effect (in comparison to one person in twenty) appears to be silver as a semi-precious metal, and silver has another advantage besides being non-irritating: it has the capacity to kill bacteria. This could be an interesting situation, and if those in the medical field were to put it across the breasts of women with possible cancer problems, it would have two effects. It would kill the bacteria, thereby eliminating the odour of perspiration, for the bacteria in perspiration is what causes it to smell. So if the bacteria is part of the breast cancer problem, then there is a chance of solving the problem without surgery and the problems associated with it.

… CHAPTER 9

Final Results—Electromagnetic Radiation

THIS INFORMATION COMES from Lyn McLean's *The Force*, in conjunction with Dr. Michael Repacholi of Adelaide Research Team.

Electromagnetic radiation and B-cell lymphomas found that radiation exposure causes the development of lymphomas B-cell and are involved in about 85 per cent of cancers. It is known that these B-cells have an important roll in the immune system.

We know that viruses are attacking our immune systems constantly, and bacteria, of course, is the cause of these diseases (Richard Loyd's *Improving the Health of Cancer Patients* is recommended reading). We know from our experiments that by putting the fabric shield in front of the power point, we can eliminate dangerous radiation and static.

We also know that the beauty of this information is that we have ways of stopping the static influence in this particular field. Now, if we go back to the centenarians, we realize that they are not in contact with our world and that they are self-sufficient and not generally in touch with people in other areas. There are people in other areas that are also long-livers, once again because they isolate themselves.

Now where are we actually going wrong? We are going wrong possibly in the fact that we are introducing to each other various types of diseases via unfamiliar bacteria or viruses. We might think that we were operating locally, but in effect, we are operating on a worldwide basis. This is emphasized particularly on aeroplanes, with people travelling from one part of the world to the other.

Why hasn't this happened to people in ancient areas? Well, to a certain extent it has. You will notice that most of the people I spoke to are single. They had been married and had their families and so forth, and then the husband generally passed on, so he somehow had an influence or had had more opportunities of being attached by outside viruses.

But how is this actually happening?? Well the biggest associated killer of, course, is the teller at the bank. Those marvellous employees are exposed to these elements all the time due to handling money. That is one big feature that this civilized world has over the ethnic groups: the civilized world handles money, and when you are talking about money, that is not only folding money (notes) but coins and credit cards too.

CHAPTER 10

The Einstein Connection

Albert's Life-and-Death Test

IN 1910, ALBERT Einstein and his partner, Conrad Harbicht, did a study in and around the town of Davos in Switzerland and concluded that there were positive and an excess of negative ions in the area. This was caused by the southerly winds that blow through Switzerland and Germany. The interesting thing is that they realized that the people were particularly healthy in these areas, to such an extent that Albert Einstein's sister, who was inflicted with tuberculosis (TB), which had been maiming and killing many people, was cured of this disease because she was treated in this area amongst all the waterfalls.

They called it electric air; we call it ionization. Amongst his friends, Albert Einstein was known as Mr Negative because of his obsession with negative ions, but you probably couldn't find anybody in the world who was more open-minded and certainly not negative in his thinking. Mr Einstein was treated respectfully. He managed to be able to measure the amount of negative ions around the rivers and got tremendous results. These, of course, would have been used to help cure his sister.

It makes you realize the power that can exist, and he conceded that the amount of negative ions could probably be 100 per cent more than he was capable of producing. When you analyse this and then consider the feng shui people of China, you'll realize that there would be thousands of locations in China, around the world, and in Europe that would have these particular geographic healing features. That is the lee side of hills nearer the bottom. The negative ion content of the water was stronger because the water was turbulent, and the more turbulence you have, the more evaporation exists. Or in other words, the greater the evaporation from water-type turmoil, the greater the amount of negative ions.

Thank you, Albert Einstein.

Einstein confirmed the Brownian movement about 1,770 years after botanist Robert Brown noticed that tiny objects like gluten grains actually moved under a microscope. Einstein confirmed that it was possible to estimate mathematically the distance that these articles should move because of molecular bombardment.

Albert Einstein proved that it is possible to actually measure a molecule and form a calculation as to what it is doing, and of course, that molecule is comprised of atoms; in turn, their condition is a by-product of a mass of ions.

We are talking about molecular bombardments when we start talking about electricity and the molecular or atomic situation of articles within the electrical or electronic world we live in. We are individually part of that electronic world, and we are actually a seething mass of molecules, electrons, and atoms, hopefully and initially designed to be in a neutral and balanced electrical state. This is not the case, in that much of the time it would be out of balance, and this is a situation when we are at risk.

This balance can be positive or negative. If the research shows as typically positive, this is not good for us. Ions in their mass and volume surround us constantly–that is, if we are lucky enough to be in a healthy environment. With a large volume of good negative ions, which are so valuable to our well being, hopefully we can try to balance the excess positive, unless the balance is too great. This explains the contented, happy attitude and brightness that you get when you are in a safe and natural environment or involved with water.

While using an electric walkway to go to the shops, some people may get an electric shock starting as low as five hundred volts and other people may not get any electric shock at all or it might take a thousand volts of static to affect them. Another fact is that it is difficult at an individual level to measure the comparison between static electricity and radiation. Obviously, it seems to me that neither of them is good. We know that static electricity is a disaster, but we don't know the level or degree of radiation in some of this static electricity. So the idea is to avoid both as much as possible, and that is very difficult when it comes to radio waves. There is strong contingent thinking that some various low frequency radio waves have a very unhealthy effect; however, the idea, of course, is to make sure that none of them get into your body, insomuch as that is possible, thus solving that problem.

We don't know what level of radiation is dangerous and personally manageable. Experts are all generalizing because we all vary—the centenarians have none, so we have some sort of starting level, and the World Health Organization says that they do not have any accurate idea because we all vary.

Consider that going back a thousand years, we theoretically weren't designed to have any imbalance at all apart from electrical storms, and of course, when that happened, people would go into caves or some other homes to protect themselves, not realizing that this had little effect in relation to their bodies. Nature was telling them to take protection, and when the storm was over, they would come out smiling happily, saying "Glad that's over" and that type of thing. Then they would go down and pick up their water or whatever, not realizing that in many instances, the new natural negative forces had actually invigorated them—they were happy. There was a degree of happiness that they thought was just the storm being over, but in effect they were being grounded in many instances, not knowing that the storm had left behind a mass of negative ions due to the fact that they were at the bottom of hills. The flow is mostly negative because the negative ions are heavier–being inhaled in balancing the massive positive and negative human electrical systems throughout the body.

Understanding Personal Body Balance
The First Line of Defence

Metal bracelets, preferably silver, will accumulate unnatural balance until the arm is grounded.

A grounded person will have a personal grounding/balance of plus or minus, yin and yang.

The cycle of grounding is completed at this point.

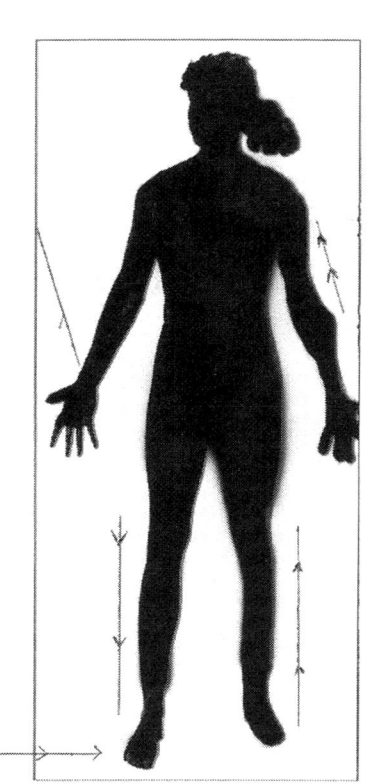

The centenarians wear jade so their bodies will absorb the minerals contained therein.

Incorrect footwear can prevent natural body balance.

Again I say thank you to Albert Einstein.

In 1932, a Dr. Hansell noticed the mood swings of a fellow scientist who worked beside an electric generator. It turned out that the machine was producing positive and negative air ions. When an adjustment was made to the machine to have it produce negative ions, this worker was happy, but when it was adjusted again back to positive, he was rude and sad. Dr. Hansel went on to produce the first ionizer.

As mentioned, Einstein's sister was cured of TB, and a chap—well recorded as having massive visible cancers—who went to the Himalayas came back cured after meditating. And then we look at Jean in her natural state, with plenty of negative ions in the home—these may not necessarily be random miracles. We should look at the possibility of expanding these results in people with diseases.

Of course, it should be noted again that in the areas that were researched, there was very little industry—even today it is used mostly for conferences and so forth. Fewer industries, of course, means fewer poisons and cleaner air. Just clarifying ionization is the omitting of electricity energy into the air, and this electricity energy actually energizes particles into the air, which those in the area then absorb.

The proof: even the old long-livers nearly always showed a small positive result on the static machine. The excess of good negative ions in the air around Davos taken via breathing and through the skin will balance out the normal existing imbalance, giving the natural exuberance that is energy excess.

These days, we can actually see what is happening to the molecules and atoms by the brilliance of new photographic techniques and the great physics experts, and they would not have had this advantage from 1910 through the 1930s.

Now, many readers might be thinking, *But that's TB; that's not my disease*, or they may be thinking, *Could it be worth a try with the disease I have?* It seems this equipment has already been made, and perhaps these modern diseases we have may require excessive positive ions to survive. If we can keep them out of the personal system, then maybe the diseases will starve or hold their ground or possibly die! Isn't it natural because it is the way we evolved from the last million years in body balance? Excesses of the heavier negative ions have been used successfully to cure other diseases as well as TB.

I will continue to proceed with this program or this theory, and it will be met with a thousand blinded-by-knowledge experts who have crossed the t's and dotted the i's all their lives. It is simple, the same as a backhand on a tennis court or a side step on a football field. It's simple when you open your mind and do it. You can't change your game unless you keep an open mind and work on it.

It cost little, instead of the tens of millions to date, and will allow the success of many near misses, which can now be reinvented and revalued by the research of the world. To put it differently, Einstein's sister was in a location where she could have constant repetitive electrical balance and negative ions. Isolation from the outside area also helped prevent the reproduction of the cause. Isn't that what all of us, diseased or healthy, are trying to do? Einstein's sister was cured of disease—and negative ion treatment has been used to treat other problems. There was also the chap in the Himalayas who was subjected to isolation and became cured; he would have been grounded also.

There are probably thirty million people with diseases such as cancer, and about half of them are close to terminal. The idea is to stop the disease and then try to cure it. If we manage to stop the disease, then the cure will follow from that by making sure that everyone is constantly grounded twenty-four hours a day, as nature intended. They can then see if the experiments are satisfactory. As it stands now, when you go to a doctor, you are loaded up with a body imbalance; you have no chance, or your chances are slim, of recovering without something being done to remedy the imbalance.

CHAPTER II

Kirlian Photography

KIRLIAN PHOTOGRAPHY IS a comparatively inexpensive way of measuring most possible diseases before they get involved permanently in your body. It is like a mini X-ray machine that works by laying your hand on a photographic plate. If you are in a good healthy state, an X-ray of your hand comes out clear and sharp. If your condition is not good, then many lines show on the Kirlian photography. They are not sharp or clear in their result, possibly due to illness or even drunkenness due to a big night out with the boys. Your hand can actually look like a gorilla's hand.

The interesting thing about this photography is that when it is applied to different parts of your hand, it indicates with lots of little lines where your body is under some form of attack or stress.

As far as I am aware, these machines are not readily available to the public—well, not here in Australia anyway—but they can be purchased online through various companies. They are called Aura Camera machines online, and they can come with an optional discharge plate. Kits are also available if you wish to make your own. These machines can be made as coin-operated machines and are much less intrusive than constant X-rays. A Professor Konstantin Korotkov has been researching their use over the past twenty-five years at St. Petersburg University. More can be read on the Web about his research.

The aim is to prevent long-term damage that gives way to diseases in various parts of your body. In other words, it's a way of having a personal warning sign of dangers that might be in the process of developing. It is quite commonly used in industry.

Another advantage of Kirlian photography is the fact that you can actually see plants being damaged and watch them deteriorate with age by the number of lines drawn in the photograph itself. It proves that the quicker you eat the vegetables after harvesting, the more energy-giving benefits exist and are retained.

The beauty of Kirlian photography is that it proves that your efforts of t'ai chi/reiki and body balance are actually working and that this whole principal is just not a matter of it "may or may not be right." You can actually see it working. It works this way: you place your hand on a plate that has electricity running through it get a nice clean definition of the plate, similar to what you would have on an X-ray.

If you were under stress, then it would show many lines as result, outlining that you are actually under stress at that time. Similarly, if you were doing your t'ai chi, you could actually see anything that was obviously wrong with you in relation to these lines. It would become very clear, and you would get a perfect reproduction of the hand.

If things are healthy in your body, the shape around the hand is nice and clean. You could even put a leaf on the plate, and it would show a perfect skeleton of the leaf. If you broke the leaf in half, you could actually see it almost as though it were bleeding, with lines going everywhere. The beauty of this is that the different positions on the hand can indicate your status immediately; you don't have to be a scientist or a doctor to understand exactly what is wrong or where your problems might be within your body.

Even concerning harmony or rage within your body, it will indicate this through the electricity coming through your hand. It also means, of course, that if your body's in perfect balance, you can see in the Kirlian plate that you are not using any necessary energy to defend yourself. You can even tell if people have had surgery, for it gives an indication of different parts of your body. It can also tell you if you are likely under attack from radicals. This could be a very handy thing to have, and they are not expensive to make. They should probably be in every railway station and every bus terminal, where for just a few dollars, people can actually evaluate themselves as to their actual conditions at a particular time. As mentioned, you can purchase one of these machines online.

Different parts of your hand represent different areas of your body and from this you can evaluate, what area needs to be checked and/or treated.

For example, the bottom of your hand represents the bowels; it would show you where possible problems might be lurking in the future. You could do it again the next day or a couple of days later and see if the problem still exists. If it does, it may be time to get a CT scan of your body, of course at a major cost, with the addition of radiation in your body –this other way gives you an idea of just where to look if you are under attack.

This has been considered similar to reflexology. It works out the fertility of seeds, the stress level of metal, and so forth. You could possibly get a little chart where it tells you where you are likely to have this problem and just relate it to your own result that you have just received on the Kirlian machine. The Germans use it quite commonly in operating theatres to confirm exactly where problems are, and they get a nice clear result in black and white, showing them the areas of problems.

Recently using Kirlian photography on the brain of a person after using a mobile phone showed massive lines in the reproduction, representing what is assumed to be EMR–electromagnetic radiation effect. We know that EMR and static can be associated together. The Winky shield, to be discussed further, along with the Brazilian experiment, confirms the cancer association.

CHAPTER 12

Understanding Meditation

THERE ARE MANY types of meditation. If conditions are right when you are walking, running, or jogging with a clean, clear mind (which is recommended before you do exercise) and you are doing it at a limit you can handle, then you can literally do these exercises without effort, and a form of meditation then exists. For this reason, think nice thoughts about happy days, loved ones, and so forth, and enjoy your walk. Keep in mind also that the walk should be purposeful, not an amble. Initially, you will be ambling as you build up condition.

The chap who went to the Himalayas would be expected to look after the group of people that he was with, which means that he would have to get up and put in the same efforts of labour. He would get himself in condition and routinely go about his activities so that he could justify the food and his very existence with these people and so forth. So his venture would not be one of just sitting in a cave. He would go about things automatically once he got used to doing what was expected of him, and he would be in a form of regular meditation. He would not be able to speak their language, so he would not get in any arguments or be a disruptive influence. No personal pressure—the avoidance of friction with people.

Later in this book we will discuss how barefooted t'ai chi people organize their meditation, and this is very important because we are going to have to do a physical split. This routine can be very important in relation to your building a reserve of energy once you have your body in balance. This reserve of energy, your grounding and personal electric balance, is your immunity against disease, backed by a strong immune system created by an increase of energy.

We now have a situation where we have to prove that the excess energy can exist. Number one is that it's strong enough to be able to fight off disease. We know that it is necessary to make sure our bodies are in balance. Electronically, we are looking as closely as we can to zero. We know that the body can be in balance, but that's not always the case, such as when we are in aeroplanes, motorcars, or what have you. So let's assume now that the body is in condition from exercise without your constantly thinking about it. You are accumulating this energy, and you are in a position now that if you were under attack, this energy would become principle in your immune system. Now how are we going to prove that such energy exists? We go to t'ai chi ch'uan.

T'ai chi is such a good, healthy thing. It gives you a higher degree of energy in reserve positively; however, let's assume the big boys come in–the big nasty diseases. By accumulating a greater chi in and around your body, t'ai chi ch'uan helps develop a reserve for your immune system. That's why some people can get an electric shock at five hundred volts, and others who run with about a thousand volts of static have a different amount of resistance to disease.

Now we get to t'ai chi ch'uan. Say a person is actually dying, as in the case of Jean, then t'ai chi ch'uan works on the principle of extreme edge. This extreme edge is serious stuff to handle. If is not done properly, it can do you more damage and kill you. Historically, many years ago this was called ultimate boxing–where you can have so much energy that you can break a person's arm just by having them push you. It is a generation of accumulated power that can be used on the sporting fields of the world. It might be something that gives a person the extra yard, extra push, drive, or the extra energy that keeps him or her alert at the right time. Many people call it accumulated adrenaline. However, let's assume you have this skill of controlled power but you don't use it as a boxing thing; you use it as a reserve. You must be in balance and condition to have this reserve.

If t'ai chi ch'uan can give you this backup reserve to have this tremendous power and you can direct it to fight against disease, then there is an excellent chance of you not getting a disease. If, however, a situation exists where your body is in electrical turmoil, like when you are in an aeroplane or sitting in your car under power lines that are leaking, then you can't defend yourself.

We need to protect and defend ourselves bodily and simply by performing exercises or walking or both. The principal is that by having both exercises in harmony, if it's snowing, raining, or a miserable night and you don't want to walk or feel it is unsafe to walk, then you can revert to t'ai chi and that energy and immune system will be waiting to be recharged. Then you are in a position to defend yourself until the weather improves. You are keeping your body in harmony, in satisfactory defence. It's as simple as that. It proves that the energy is your saviour, your immune system balanced since with its unnatural static imbalanced electricity has been involved in the world—this modern world. With all the benefits that televisions, computers, and other great things that electricity gives you, you have to be on top of it. You have to be in physical control, and this will give you just that so you'll have a substantial energy level following the example of the t'ai chi using the Okinawans' method.

With that strength and expanded immune system, if no problems exist, you are still in a situation where you are in control. It's similar to the soccer goalkeeper's alert action, ready to step into the game. If you are in a serious situation and time's limited, then you have a chance of calling on these reserves, the immune system (hopefully already in action) and that energy. You don't feel it, of course, and it's not as though you can just pull it in. It means you do have the capacity, with determination and a mental attitude of letting your body know that it's not over till it's over, using all resources. Believe you're winning. Remember the feng shui way that ancients drew trees on their walls when none were around and the current so-called new thinking—good as it is—of thinking positively to help cure yourself. It works- we are probably about a thousand years behind the ancient thinking.

This transition starts when you are a young person, and you continue with this practice of walking or jogging and keeping the t'ai chi going in conjunction with it. The advantage of doing this is that you're not getting diseases, whether it's a simple cold, flu, or normal sickness that we all get, which is the ageing thing, and then you can continue being younger than your years. So when you hit one hundred years old, you will only look seventy and will have the strength and complexion of a seventy-year-old, like the Okinawans. Eat the right foods and the idea is that when you are forced to change from your lifestyle because of circumstances or economy or you are meant to retire at a certain age, your routine will change but not necessarily your t'ai chi. That will keep your body in tune, for your body will be expecting it. With your new ventures, maybe it's going kayaking at an older age, you're still doing your t'ai chi and expecting that your body is creating a new energy-developing exercise. You're tricking your body by keeping 50 per cent of it in your system; your body is expecting that. Therefore, you are creating an age gap between your true age and your deteriorating age, which is nothing like it should be when comparing it with your previous energy.

This, of course, has a great advantage for the oldies of the world. There is no reason that by using this knowledge, they can't extend their 100 or 110 years to a much greater age. Because they will be starting back further down the line, the same as you are right now. It works. It's worked for them, and there is no reason that it can't work for us in the Western world as well.

If you actually have a disease, this is your best defence. Otherwise, there may be very little hope for you. It changes the rules of engagement, if you like, and you will have a chance of living a normal life, everything being as it should, for some period anyway.

CHAPTER 13

Stress Proteins

MARVELLOUS AND VALUABLE research is being done by the scientists who are busy crossing the t's and dotting the i's on stress proteins, now called heat shock proteins in the Western world. They generalize and emphasize the fact that under stress, various proteins expand or open and close to try to balance any stress situation existing in the human body. Millions of dollars have been spent on determining what chemicals are activated within the human body for this reaction to take place, and the Western way of knowing every detail as to why this is so only confuses the situation, which was solved a hundred or perhaps a thousand years previously.

Stress is worry that when retained in your mind tends to grow and grow. This can cause anxiety and depression, which in some cases can be difficult to override. We need to have diversions to take our minds off the problem(s) and to make our bodies feel relaxed. The centenarians do this with a constant routine of everyday tasks and relaxing on the weekend when the family comes to visit. We need to get those happy endorphins released in our brains.

One of the fundamental features when comparing the centenarians, the guy in the Himalayas, the one who travelled around Australia (said to be hearsay), us on the yacht, and Mum and Jean is the fact that in almost every case where there has been contact with other people, it has been happy. Where there were decisions to make, they were made largely by a group. I mention here the council, the Layisus, the Okinawans, and the women who were heading for the sugar farm—everything done as a group.

In the future, application of this amazing research will help millions of people, but unfortunately for those dying of some of these diseases now, it is not going to help a great deal. But what does help us a great deal is the final result that the people of hundreds of years ago have achieved and that is helpful in giving them this extended life. They do this by avoiding stress. Scientists have given us magic details of how it works—the principal of what we individually are involved in on a day-to-day basis is to make sure that this stress doesn't apply.

Nothing applies but lack of stress, and stress is happening by having contact with other people and their problems, like every time the telephone rings. This is important because it depends on a mental attitude here. Every time the telephone rings, you might think, *Well, there's a problem.* But it's not a problem; it is a solution that has to be solved, and it can be a positive.

Talking to a euthanasia group can also help relieve stress levels, as happened in the case of Jean, and we believe it did help extend her life. It may or may not necessarily mean you are interested in becoming involved in euthanasia, but just knowing help is available can relieve so much tension and anxiety.

The Dalai Lama, when asked what surprised him most about humanity, answered, "Man. Because he sacrifices his health in order to make money. Then he sacrifices money to recuperate his health. And then he is so anxious about the future that he does not enjoy the present; the result being that he does not live in the present or the future; he lives as if he is never going to die, and then dies having never really lived."

I can proudly say that Jean really *lived*.

CHAPTER 14

Apartment Living

IF YOU GROW your own vegetables, then you are aware of their history. You know what you have used to fertilize them, and that you have used natural and safe means to keep them disease-free and so forth. As said many times throughout this book, we should eat as *freshly* and *naturally* as possible.

Living in an apartment does not have to stop us from doing this. You can get a flat pan/dish/pot approximately two inches in height. If you wish, it can have dividers to separate your different types of seeds. Place a thin layer of cotton wool in the bottom and sprinkle a reasonable amount of seeds to create your own veggie patch with optimum vitamins similar to the Okinawans' long life grass. Make sure you keep the cotton wool damp. This way, you can have vegetables that can be grown out of season because they are being grown indoors.

Caring for these vegetables/herbs/seeds is easy. Just locate them near a window where there is plenty of light and sun and you can harvest them as needed simply by cutting the tops off with scissors when they reach around three inches in height. They will be there to go into your next salad or dish—preferably left uncooked. These mini gardens can look quite attractive, and at any time you can transfer them to an outside garden by processing them into a potting mixture. Some of the many herbs available for this type of planting are basil, thyme, balm, chives, coriander, dill bouquet, summer savory, rosemary, and many more. Don't forget the *chomeigusa*, the Okinawan long life grass.

Many years ago, my sailing partner George and I sailed double-handed from Melbourne to Osaka in a yacht race. We had an unfortunate explosion in the engine compartment, and it left us without power when we got into the Northern Hemisphere, north of the equator, and one of the side stays holding up the mast almost broke in a storm. We realized that if we took on any load on the portside in relation to wind, we were going to lose our mast, which would mean we could not steer in the direction that we intended. We had to "run off," as they say in the yachting world, to take load off that side of the rig. Without power, radio, lights, water pumps, and communication, a serious situation existed in relation to being adrift without help. Prior to leaving Melbourne and having knowledge of the health of plants, we actually set up a situation where we caught rainwater and used the same principals as above to grow food. When we eventually got to Osaka in Japan via Sextant, our physical condition was good. The only fresh food we had had was our plants and lentils, which we snipped off to add to our meals. Captain Cook found out many years ago the importance of fresh food when he discovered eastern Australia. We did have a dramatic weight loss that could be of interest to some readers—George and I used mostly wheat grass.

Another aid for healthy living in an apartment is to be aware that if you think polluted air may be coming into your area, you don't leave your windows open to allow pollutants to enter. As mentioned previously, you could install a wind-indicating device, and these are available from most marine equipment suppliers. This would indicate the path of the possible pollutants and allow you to choose unaffected windows where this polluted draft/breeze cannot reach. Be aware.

Alternatively, you could also install an air purifier. They are not expensive and are much cheaper than having bad health and the costs associated with it. Leave the windows open if the air is good. My idea of bad air is air that is coming from distant coal-fired power stations, as the residue carries mercury poisons. If this situation exists, just close the windows and put on your air purifier. Some purifiers also have antibacterial filters. If you're in category two (your disease is serious) or three (your disease is terminal), consider equipment that makes these good negative ions.

We individually have to look at our homes. We spend about half of our lives in our homes, and we have to make sure that they are as safe as we can possibly be from the point of static electricity in relation to our lifestyles.

We did not know what we were doing with Jean. The first thing we did, because of business experience, was put plants at the front door of the house and at the back door of the house so that you couldn't get in or out of the house without coming into contact with a plant. You also need the same situation near your toilet. Frankly, you cannot have too many plants in your house that you are going to brush past.

Feng shui people did not know about electronics, but they always point out that you should have a tree in your house. They did not realise that what they were actually doing was earthing themselves in their homes. We know the power of the human mind concerning personal healing. Was this tree painting a positive healing effect, tricking their minds because they knew the strength of trees? They and the ancients were hundreds of years in advance–simply thinking from a different square, like most of this book. This is important these days, and we understand that if you think positively, you get a better result. There are many ways of doing these things personally. For example, if you have a metal towel rack set right beside a single bed so that if you rolled over in bed and touched that towel rack, you would be immediately grounded, and there are many other clever things you can work into your own little world.

Understand when you walk into your home what the situation is in relation to flooring. There is no doubt that going barefoot is best, but it's not always feasible because of the cold.

Make sure your socks and your shoes are suitable in relation to your carpet. In addition to the socks, we need the carpet to be natural (i.e., wool or cotton). Remember that cotton is the best product in your house, as you don't want static building up because you are using the wrong fabrics and so forth. Likewise, as far as getting negative ions into the house, the television is not good for that. We do know that if you feel air around your room, even if it is coming from a fan, that new air being circulated will help against the ions being stolen by the television and possibly computers to some extent.

Don't forget that at night it is also necessary for you to have a circulation of clean air around you all the time. You should be able to feel a breeze—adjust the window so that you do get that breeze. Blankets that you can positively breathe through allow that circulation as part of your immune system. Cotton blankets with aerating capabilities are now used in Western hospitals—use them on your home beds. I am currently writing to the Australian Wool Board to see if they can manufacture such a product to match the expensive mohair and so forth that exist in the market place. I will be making regular reports regarding the results that I get from these endeavours.

CHAPTER 15

Daily Routines to Maintain Health

FIRSTLY, GO TO bed one hour earlier and get up one hour earlier to walk, jog, swim, or what have you. You will personally have to access the variations to suit your own particular lifestyle.

Now let's take a reconstructed hypothetical day. You wake up in the morning and make a toilet stop. You have brushed past your plant, which has given you a grounding feature. You have worn clothes that are generally or usually cotton; you had no synthetic clothes on you, so you have a reasonable balance statically, although not perfect. We will give you ways to make it perfect in the future–watch the website. Hop into the shower and do at least two types of exercises whilst in there. This is quite important–we need repetitiveness, and this is one of the keys to success, as mentioned. So you want to be able to effortlessly do exercises that you are going to use in your work. Let's say that your job is to pack shelves, which means you are constantly going to squat down and move along a bit. You repeat your actions until you have finished the whole row of shelves. That is exhausting, but had you done exercises similar to the actions that you are now using, then you would have accumulated a great deal of unused energy. An example of that is the Japanese people—they sit on the floor, they jump up and down as though it were nothing, and their bodies are twisted in an unusual shape as they fold their legs underneath them, but it is all natural to them. They are not using any energy because their bodies are conditioned to it.

You can talk to a physio or a chap who specialises in exercises. Most clubs have them, and they can recommend an exercise that you can do it in the shower in relation to other exercises that you are likely to have had recommended to you. It is not a matter of what the government says you must do or that it is all about the exercises that *you* need. And once you do these exercises, they can give you pleasure as you feel yourself getting fit. You can go out for half an hour in your little kayak that you might have down on the water, just as long as you are getting repetitive exercise that is not exhausting.

You have now done your exercises in the shower and have been for walk or a swim and one of the exercises that you may not have been able to do if the weather has been unfavourable. It's time to get yourself dressed. It is important that the shoes that you are going to wear to work have leather soles or heels. Make sure that the socks that you are wearing are cotton, for cotton is semi-conductive, and hopefully the innersole is conductive as well so that you have natural electricity going right through you from your feet to the ground.

You may be going to work by bus or your car to a bus stop. If going via car, note that for about ten dollars, you can put a static strap on the back of the car—now theoretically everybody in that car is earthed when getting into it, as long as the person isn't wearing staticky clothes. As mentioned, this can happen very quickly so make sure that you are wearing cotton underpants and clothing. If you have leather seats, then you typically needn't worry.

You get out of the car and race to the station, sometimes running late, perhaps because your kids are not keeping up to scratch with timing. Now, if you have incorporated your jogging exercises, then that thirty-yard run to the train line or bus line won't leave you puffing or blowing because you are well practiced. You get onto the bus and see that it is full. There are no seats, so you will have to hold on to a support strap. Usually these things can be plastic, synthetic rubber, or whatever and you don't know whether you will be grounded or not, so if there is one of those steel poles going up to the roof, hold on to that or grip something metal, and that will ground you for your trip.

It wouldn't cost the bus company any more than it cost you to put the static strap on your car, so tell the bus driver that you want a static strap on that bus! If he doesn't have it in the next couple of days, ask him why he hasn't spoken to the boss about it. Explain to him that he is in health trouble too.

You get into the lift feeling fit because your exercises have been going well. Moreover, you have recently read Dale Carnegie's book *How to Win Friends and Influence People*–the best book I have ever read–and when you relate it to this book and practice it, you will feel that it probably should have been called *How to Avoid Stress*. You are smiling at everyone with a daily greeting. Everyone is happy, and it is almost contagious. As you smile at others, you look them in the eye. If there is a woman in a different department who has been giving you a bit of a snarl, think of something that is nice about her–even if just the quality of her blouse or a change of her hairstyle–and make a comment: "You are looking good." Be friendly and break the ice. Don't necessarily take it any further–just make friendly eye contact and speak the truth.

Put in as good a day's work as you possibly can. When you get out of the lift, brush by the plants that you asked the boss to put in and keep in mind that they have to be watered, making sure that they are in good health. It's possibly best to have ferns and plants that do not have flower because you don't want pollen in the atmosphere around you.

Have a talk to your boss about getting a reading of persons' electrical balance in that room in which you are working. It may cost him some money, and he may object to or say it is not worthwhile, but it is not a lot of money when you consider the increase in productivity that he will get from people who are alert and in balance. If your boss does not give you a favourable response, then perhaps you could purchase one yourself for your own particular area, as the cost is very little. Remember to mention that it is healthier for the boss as well as yourself, with fewer people having sick days. Another way of putting it to him is that he could hire the equipment or buy one unit for the whole floor or the whole building, depending on the size, and do it in areas where you are getting good electrical balance with the people. My statistics with the people I am working with: There is one person in four in very bad balance, and these are the people at risk. At this time, you can turn them on to the principles in this book and lend them the book to show them how they can get healthier and have a chance of dodging the radicals.

Knock off time. You decide to have a beer with friends—it is good as an un-winder! My mum always had a brandy with dry ginger ale at night before she went to bed. Jean always had at least two glasses of wine. She seemed to have a limit of two—one when she was cooking and one with dinner. Don't forget that the Hunzas have wine also.

Try to avoid friction with your loved one. Give everybody a kiss when you come home to get things started on the right foot. Try to be interested in how they are getting along, regardless of how tired you feel. If feeling stressed, then this might be a good time to take a shower—a grounding exercise!

Evaluate everything you do. Are you doing everything the safest way to keep yourself grounded? Put yourself in the same situation as the Hunzas, where they are isolated from the rest of the world and try to do that as far as possible in your own home or business.

If you have the opportunity to get a Karlian reading and you believe you are in the category one situation, then certainly at least once a week make sure you get a reading of how you are doing. If you are in the two or three bracket, then it would be a good idea at least every second day to have a reading–keep those lines clear and clean. Eat what the specialists in the food department recommend.

You now want to go to the local storekeeper and buy some goods. The storekeeper has employed the new recommended cash register drawers to their electronic machines, which has killed all the germs, and that change has been transferred to you without any bacteria because it has all been killed. So all radicals, including cancer, bacteria, or viruses, that could have existed prior are now destroyed. We have to give this particular treatment a name. We will call it the Parana. This will be our registered name that will allow both the person using the drawer and the customer to know that their products/change is safe. It will have an extension as well–an additional system devised by Norwood Cash Drawers Systems, which will have a way of protecting the operator by the technique, allowing the operator to be grounded all the time as well as providing protection to and from the person handling the money in relation to diseases. So that way, the operator and the customer are disease-free from the transaction. The purpose is to avoid foreign bacteria through both money and static balance—aiming for radiation control personally.

On the way home, try to get fresh air as much as possible. Trains are bad news in relation to the amount of negative ions that are destroyed. Try to keep your head away from any engine, be it electrical, manual, or diesel.

The Danger of Power Points

When you come into your house, be aware that you can get both a static and a radiation charge if you are within two feet nine inches, according to our measurements, from electrical power points. (See page 103.) Keep as clear as you can from that. Grounding is important so that you don't get any accumulation of any voltage within your body. Again—no shoes in the house.

CHAPTER 16

Bridget, Jason, Ben, and Don

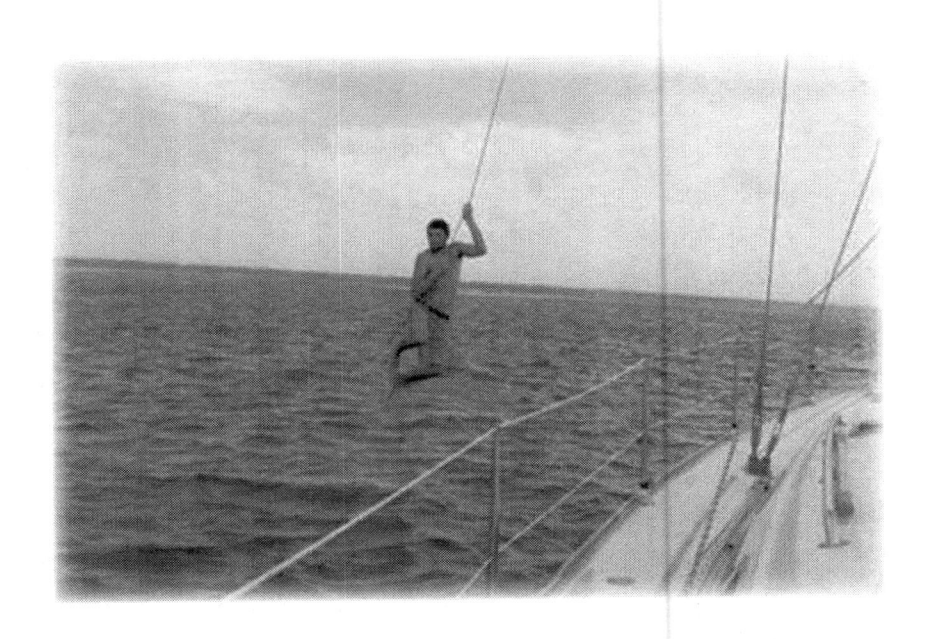

The effect of negative ions!
Could any disease survive or match this energy?

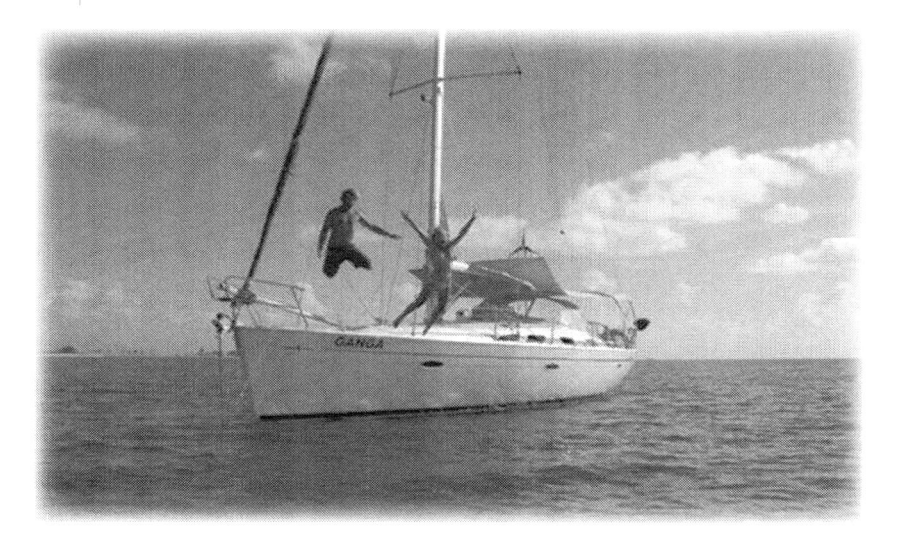

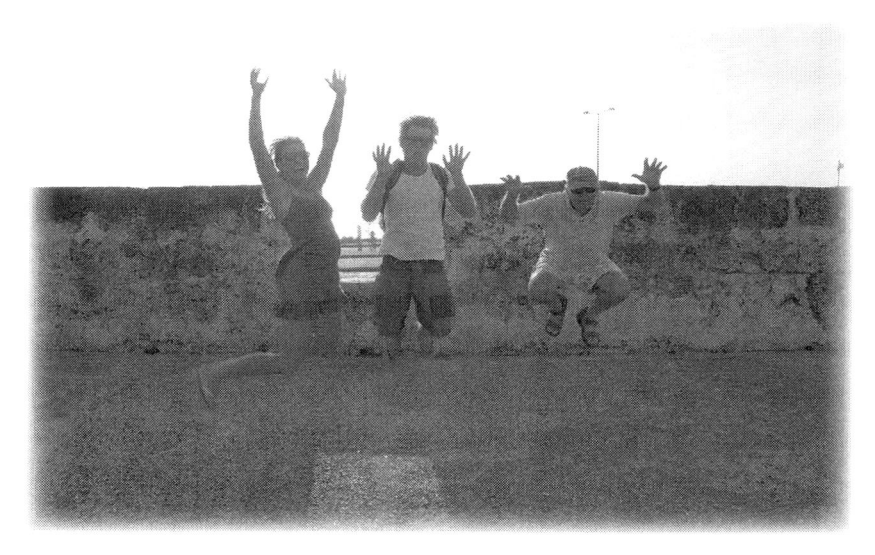

The result of excess energy!

ON THE YACHT, we had exceeded the balance of electricity stability within the body even better than any of the others tested because we were surrounded by water, which means we were all grounded and stress-free.

Being in the state of *constant* body balance could have a dramatic effect on all our futures. My idea was that diseases live off positive content. The energy created by any excess of negative ions, as our reading showed whilst on the boat, would give us the ability to fight off disease. Obviously, we have to get near balance, but what would happen if we could actually generate tremendous negative ions even greater than that minus four volts that was the maximum we got out on the sailing trip? Is it worth investigating? You will tear this book up if you let my imagination run riot here and say that perhaps it's the secret of nearly eternal life. Please don't do so—remember that it was Albert Einstein who said, "Imagination is more important than knowledge."

Seriously, I hope that after we have published this book, it will help progress along these lines. This is how we finished up after the trip, in my opinion, stable with more negative in our system, which was verified by the consistency of the negative boat results of all of us; and we put ourselves—and Jean put herself—in a situation of close to perfect health as far as constant body balance is concerned.

CHAPTER 17

Food and Diet

THE VEGETABLES WE buy from the stores are typically around five days to over a week in age, so you are really eating a dying product. Should these vegetables be certified organically grown and/or snap frozen and eaten quickly when harvested, you have an excellent chance of building up a good energy balance.

Relate this to the old people of the world, the centenarians, who look as though they are many years younger. You also have the distinct advantage of getting the benefits of eating freshly grown veggies. All ethnic groups would just go pick their vegetables for dinner, probably every night or every second night. The people of Bama would just walk across their bridge and select what they felt like for a meal, and the Okinawans would go and collect their herbs, wildly grown, and their vegetables that they had grown themselves.

A researcher, Paavo Airola, PhD, referred to correct food as the secret of life itself. The fresher the plant or the greener, the greater the power to duplicate. We are referring to the reproductive power as energy. That is exactly the same thing, but he refers to it as the secret of life itself. Also he points out very astutely that they concentrate on the foods that they have traditionally eaten. For example, they don't look for foreign foods if they are eating beans, alfalfa, wheat, and soya beans. You don't try to force milk on them if that is not one of their basic products. However, if you were in Australia or America, you would probably consider milk if it didn't upset you as part of a staple in your diet.

Mr. Airola divides the food into different sections. It says that seeds, nuts, and grains are very powerful and goes on to talk of vegetables and fruits. Once again, all eaten as raw and as young as possible. Mr. Airola's book *How to Get Well* is worth a read.

Compare the denatured food, refined food, or man-made foods that you get from stores against the natural foods grown without fertilizers or chemicals and sprays. Mr. Airola made a valuable comment when he said that breakfast foods are denatured foods: toxic preservatives and white sugar are some of the additives. This comes from the refining of white flour, where he says that twenty valuable nutrients exist before they are enriched; only four nutrients remain and are returned to the refined product. Breakfast cereals are a perfect example of this, as is white bread. Let's draw a comparison here to the survival rate of Jean and her breakfast of fruit and porridge with brown sugar; she always had a cup of tea as well. You can do a lot with porridge by compounding it and making it into a biscuit (such as the Hunzas do). When you add fluid, you're back to porridge. When you realize the high nutrient value of natural food, it's obvious that you just don't need as much food. This will affect any potential weight problems, and you will have the same amount of or more energy throughout the day.

Processed food is becoming our biggest killer. We don't know what we are eating. Governments are coming along and saying certain levels are good enough. They don't appreciate that we all vary. Some people can take one level of poison and it won't hurt them, whereas another person can have the same level and it makes him or her physically upset. This food business is one of trying to eat as naturally as you can and eating less out of packets while mimicking what the centenarians do.

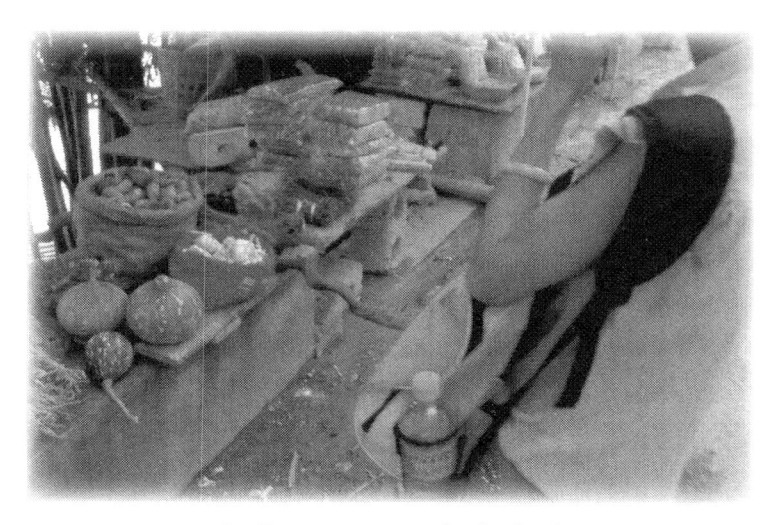

In Bama–super fresh foods
(Note jade bracelet on left arm)

CHAPTER 18

Exercise

WE NOW GET this information from the computer, which shows the worst and best possible situation with ions. Relate now how healthy you feel when you walk through the forest (or the bush, as we call it in Australia), along the beaches near water, and amongst the trees. Where there is high ion content, consider the situation where the body is in balance. You're earthed and right back with nature. You feel alive and full of energy because that's what it is actually giving you. You are building up your energy level. You can't feel alive unless you have energy. Energy is your counter-attack against disease. Although she had a disease, Jean was physically active. Although she was dying, she could play a game of golf and still finish the full eighteen holes.

When she read that Greg Norman used metal golf clubs instead of graphite, she used the metal ones—constantly unknowingly grounding herself. When she was feeling off, she would get a golf cart, but I never saw her once where she wasn't fit enough to complete a round. Through this constant exercise, she looked as though the dying had stopped—and she acted like it had too!

CHAPTER 19

Air Travel and Associated Problems and Possible Solutions

SAY WE ARE in a position where, because of the situations we are in—which could be aeroplanes, motor cars, hospitals, air conditioning, badly ventilated premises, or what have you—all of a sudden our static levels have gone berserk, as they did in Bama with the centenarian and they did with Jason and me on the aeroplane when we went to the Caribbean. This is not an easy situation to find yourself in, for the body is in absolute turmoil, and of course, as we know, static is an accumulative thing, so we actually have to find a way of balancing that, preferably before it happens. We know that our bodies will usually show a predominately electrically positive result even if marginally out of balance. A way of stopping this could be to make sure there are enough negative ions created to get those bodies back into balance if we can't do it by grounding ourselves. However, we are in a position to actually manufacture products that create negative ions, and if we can get those negative ions into our systems, then we can automatically have a neutral balance by the negative ions balancing out the excess of the positives that usually exist within our bodies.

I am working to create a product where you can know every time your body is out of balance, and we know now how to get ourselves back into balance by grounding ourselves, but this may not always be possible, such as when on aeroplanes. Nevertheless, as long as the accumulation of static is not too great, then we can make negative ions in enough proportions to actually counteract this positive feature throughout our bodies, giving us electrical stability. It would be very easy and economical for the passengers moving onto a plane to ground themselves before they started their flight. It would cost virtually nothing if they just followed simple procedures of grounding themselves before they went through the tunnel and onto the plane.

Until recently, this problem was initially solved for the passengers by their having to walk to their flight on the tarmac. The attendants would wheel a portable stepladder to the entry into the plane, and they would have carry-on baggage in one hand as they climbed the stairs. There was always a rail for them to hang on to, and it was always made of metal. This would ground the people getting onto that plane, and they would start their journey in a grounded position. But it does not mean that the static wouldn't accumulate—the speed of the plane would obviously accumulate static, as speed is a static creator. It's the same with cars and trains, but at least they are starting at a basic zero level. This procedure no longer exists on these modern planes with the smart walkways and so forth.

I have written to the principals of Boeing and probably the world's safest airline, Qantas, letting them know of the situation that exists. We know that they will come back and say that they have the world's purest air, but they haven't; they couldn't have for me to get the results that I have spoken of. They couldn't have assessed the electrical balance or static level of their customers. They would automatically have in their wing tips anti-static equipment to protect the plane. There is no doubt that they would have to have that same anti-static situation around the pilots to protect the electronics in the plane, and would have a backup if there was too much static in that cockpit.

The thing of course that is not considered a scenario could exist where there is so much static in the back of the plane, including the passenger build-up, and if that static were to be carried through to the cockpit, it could cause massive electrical malfunctions with the instruments as a result of these high static zones. There is usually no way of physically hand steering many of these modern planes if that did happen, in spite of their backup systems, as many of the new planes cannot be flown mechanically any more. I mention again that I am in the electronics field.

So it would make a good scenario for a movie perhaps, but it is certainly worth considering that the people in the plane haven't been considered as far as electronics, in spite of their promises of good clean air. We know that if a person is out of balance, then he or she is open to diseases! It is as simple as that. So we hope we get a satisfactory response from these organizations, these manufacturers. Their interest will be reported to the people via the various websites, which will give their responses. They are going to have to take some action after reading this!

The thing that should also be considered here is the fact that with me starting our trip at two volts and Jason starting at nine volts, what about those people who are starting their trip with what is supposed to be the Westerners' average of forty volts! As static levels accumulated, they would be off the planet. What about those people, and there might be some of them on the plane, who can get an electrical shock just going up an escalator when going to the stores to do their shopping? They must be running at a minimum rate of five hundred volts, and if they start accumulating at the same rate that we accumulated ours, then we have people in very serious electrical situation. With the ordinary negative ions that would rarely exist on a plane at any satisfactory volume, due to air conditioning, there is no way for the positive electricity in the body to be balanced out.

When that situation exists, as has been previously proven by other research, these diseases are being created by bacteria or viruses—and these people that you are flying with, maybe in a very close proximity to yourself, are actually transiting diseases, leaving you totally defenceless unless your reserves of energy supporting your immune system are enough to counter the attack.

We don't know what reserves of energy are required to meet such a situation. There is a study that has been done by Richard Loyd, PhD, which says that most cancers are not medical emergencies that required immediate invasive and toxic interventions—it is a degenerative condition that requires improving of health. Jean was an example of this.

As mentioned above, the speed of the plane obviously accumulates static speed, as speed is a static creator. It should be noted, for example, that in an aircraft travelling at thirty thousand feet, it's usually an efficient height with low atmospheric conditions existing at that altitude and can acquire a plane body voltage of one million volts or more, and this obviously impacts the passengers. While the plane is designed to handle such a problem, can we say the same thing about humans?

We have seen photographs of petrol stations being ignited by persons carrying too much electricity in their bodies when getting out of their motor vehicles, causing fires and serious health risks.

In Belgrade in May 2000, a Beechcraft exploded due to the handler having too much electricity in his body when he was refuelling the plane. There was also a recognized suspicion that the deaths of 250 people that occurred on the TWA flight from New York to Paris in 1996 may have been the result of static electricity. That doesn't make the film scenario such a wild possibility.

The mentioning of these problems is not to frighten people about flying; there are too many planes in the sky to consider your survival from something being wrong with the plane quite unlikely. With training and ideas improving all the time, you are in safe hands, but it does clarify the situation of the people inside the planes in relation to their health and their defensive mechanisms having any reasonable effect at all because of the situation of static at the time of the flight. Of course, I am offering my services to the various airlines in an effort to create a better chance of survival in this electronic world.

It also should be noted at this particular point that many famous sports and political people seem to have an abnormal amount of rogue diseases in spite of their tremendous physical capabilities and obviously their energy storage, or chi, if you are an Asian reading this. These people are travellers, and they travel around the world to meet their sporting and business obligations. Of course, this could have been the cause of my wife getting her disease, as she did a vast amount of travelling. As far as the grounded oldies of the world, including my 104-year-old mum and the oldies of Bama, Okinawa, and so forth, who have done very little travelling, I feel that because they did not or do not travel but stay with their own groups, not mixing with outsiders, they are not subjected to the diseases carried by outsiders.

It should be noted that Jean got on that plane with undiagnosed liver cancer, *but* it only became evident when she went on board and was surrounded by the lack of good negative ions, largely due to the air conditioning and the fact that she could not be grounded because she was on a plane. Would Albert Einstein–Mr. Negative–have said that this was "just a coincidence"?

When talking about static, airlines could and should take into account the type of fabrics and furnishings used on the aircraft and possibly making use of natural products, such as cotton, informing their cliental of the health benefits of non-static clothing.

Malaysian airlines have had a problem since I began writing this book, and the possibility of static electricity being involved was not considered.

Boeing Brisbane, Australia, has not replied to my letter.

If you are obliged to do an aeroplane trip, then this is the procedure that I would follow knowing what I know now. I would first make sure that I was grounded before I went into the airport. Find a metal pole or something metal to touch; hopefully if it is unpainted, it will be conductive electrically. Of course, when you go into the airport to do your ticketing, do it as automatically as you can, keeping away from people handling your tickets. Always be sure you're wearing a long cotton shirt in case you have to sit next to a person you don't know–you don't want physical contact. You don't know where the person's bacteria may have come from. Before you get onto the plane, go to the toilet and dry your hands with a paper towel. Don't throw the paper towel away, and as you exit the toilet facility when you open the door, make sure the paper towel is between you and the door handle.

The door will always open towards you, and the door will have hundreds of people's germs on it. Find the closest bin and discard the paper towel. If you are on one of those automatic walkways, see if you can find something metal to touch with the back of your hand.

When you get onto the plane again, if you have a choice, try to have as many stops as you can rather than doing it all in one flight. When you go to the toilet again, try to keep the voltage down and try to handle some metal somewhere on the plane. If you are a flight attendant, and if you are handing metal plates of food around, make sure you touch the metal on the plate for grounding purposes (but I guess these days much of the dinnerware is plastic, or china if travelling in first class).

If you are constantly covered in an electronic field, such as in the case of checkout staff, and you are a woman, the idea of the fabric shield across your breast would probably be a good one if you have breast problems or have areas where you have cancer. Look at the idea of having the fabric shield being put over these areas. You must understand that this is an amazing product. It feels like silk. If it was put into a slot across your breast, then you can be assured that every test that we have personally done has made your breasts protected from radiation and static. The idea is to have it slotted as a link from breast to breast.

CHAPTER 20

Carcinogenic Products

THE INTERNATIONAL AGENCY for Research on Cancer, the IARC, classifies carcinogens that are positively carcinogenic to humans. Levels of exposure are often hundreds of times higher than any exposure people experience from daily use of consumer products. Carcinogenic means cancer creating.

Now different countries have different standards in relation to how much of this dangerous product is allowed in the manufacture of their products, but what we should note here is that as with static electricity, some people require as low as five hundred volts to get an electric shock when going up an escalator and some people require one thousand volts, as mentioned previously in the book. The fact is that people do vary also in their levels of resistance in relation to energy or chi reserves. The old people of the world have none of these products, so who is to determine what a safe level is? The level of safety is zero and should remain at zero if you want to have an extended life.

It should also be noted that of all the different ethnic groups that I tested, their homes were, without exception, at least thirty years old, sometimes probably one hundred years old, and any products used in their construction, such as glues, asbestos, particle board, and so on, that may have existed as far back as thirty-odd years before have dissipated from the environment they live in.

We know that gasoline is carcinogenic, as are some preservatives, fertilizers, insecticides, and so forth. A full list is available on the Web. Should it become necessary to use some of these pollutants, then a mask should be worn to protect one from inhaling these dangerous substances or pollutants. It is notable that the oldies' homes were always situated a fair distance away from the roads to avoid breathing in fumes. There was an exception at Layisu, where the main road ran through the town, but there is very little traffic because the area is so remote.

A synthetic product called formaldehyde is involved in 85 per cent of all cancers. Remember the 85 per cent recorded carcinogenic content of formaldehyde, making the possibility of the result highly predictable. Now, with solutions and means to attack from the civilized viewpoint and an immediate solution for afflicted smokers by destroying the carcinogenic factor; as a parallel, we have the knowledge of how to destroy the bad static factor and keep the personal electrical balance in the system as it was meant to be, naturally. We have the knowledge now to destroy the static factor and perhaps radiation content.

An experiment involving nicotine and formaldehyde should be undertaken to see if the combined formula causes cancer or whether a third catalyst/situation such as body imbalance is required. As I write this, I cannot find any past experiments regarding this situation, but you would think that it may have been done somewhere in the past. Information would help, please. The experiment would be comparatively inexpensive by today's standards and would need to be carried out by a chemist, as I do not have the qualifications required, but with help from people who will support this book, it would be a worthwhile experiment. This means, of course, that once we know what articles/products have this particular substance in them (and as mentioned, it should be banned worldwide), we then may be in a position to eradicate many of these diseases happening in the first place.

We believe old lawn bowls contain the use of formaldehyde in their manufacture. Therefore, we should enlist the help of these manufacturers to produce a bowl that is free from this substance—unless this problem has already been solved. Simply ask the manufacturers if this is the case. The bowl-cleaning rags can also carry contamination and should not be carried into your home. Without destroying the lawn bowl industry, we feel a way could be found to protect the bowlers and their families, perhaps with the use of a disposable cloth and receptacle to destroy them and their containments.

This research comes from Greenpeace on the situation of teas, including Jasmine teas, black teas, and green teas coming from China. The research showed that all eighteen samples taken contained at least three pesticides, with seven pesticides found in the worst sample. The pesticides included such things as methomyl and endosulfan, which have been banned by the World Health Organisation as being dangerous to health. Another bad one was fenvalerate, which can cause harm to unborn children and can cause genetic damage. These pesticides have been banned internationally. The logical suggestion, of course, is to not drink these Chinese teas until they get their act together. Unfortunately, it creates suspicion in what you are drinking from other tea manufacturers. Let's hope the Greenpeace organisation continue their investigations in this regard internationally. The only solution seems to be to drink only organically produced teas or teas produced in high-altitude regions that don't need pesticides because of their growing conditions.

CHAPTER 21

Recommendations for the Building Industry

MANY OF THE resins and toxic materials that exist in the building industry affect the homes, hospitals, and so forth, in which modern people reside. They are usually poorly aerated with few windows, affecting people physically. This may be another of the reasons that the old people of the world who do not have these particular products in the construction of their own homes have the advantage of not being poisoned by our civilized world. Again, this could explain why their own people who move out of the old environments and their established homes, away from the old ways and the old farming methods and into the moneymaking world of civilization, become more susceptible to disease. They had greater health benefits before moving and entering this new world of poisons.

For us in this Western world we live in, it's virtually impossible to stop and change our ways, but putting plenty of good air through our world and diluting these poisons will help. The old people of the world typically get plenty of ventilation through their windows because they usually aren't constructed as tightly as most windows, allowing natural amounts of air, the same as in Jean's and my home.

If I were building a house or premises in the future and wanted magnificent flooring materials, I would get a response in writing as to the origin/composition and treatment needed as well as method and materials used in the laying of the floor—glue and so forth.

As well as the resin holding particleboards together, which is a VOC, some other sealants in the house, such as stains, latex-based paints, and so forth, may exist and will last for years. Other dangerous toxins include xylene and products containing methylene chloride, benzene, and so on. Most, like formaldehyde, are carcinogenic (i.e., cancer-creating products).

In every case, it is recommended to have lots of ventilation—masses of air through the building to dilute any toxins contained therein, and on its completion, don't rush into the new house. Wait some weeks if possible and air diligently. As said previously, VOCs can last for years, but of course, it is not feasible to wait for years before you enter your new home, so you have to be constantly airing your dwelling as much as possible.

If you apply the advantages of a degree of negative ions trying to help build up your immune system, then it makes more sense to be as physically strong and as in balance as possible.

It is true that we are representing the negative ions as being the good ions because they are heavier; therefore, when a split occurs, the positives stay high because they are physically lighter in weight. However, I should mention that when you are watching television, the negative ions are attracted to the picture and the positive ions are left behind and not helping the positive and negative body balance at the human ground level. Again, the solution is plenty of fresh air in the room. If you are using the television and other electrical units, then this gets the new flow of negative ions through the atmosphere of the area.

Here is a list of the poisons that are commonly used in the building industry. The US Environmental Protection Agency has identified sixteen thousand of them under concern. Other serious products are vinyl, which is the most widely used plastic polymer in the United States. Then there is PVC in many forms, chlorinated plastics, diaoxins, and chlorine. Dioxins include some of the most carcinogens know to humankind, affecting the immune system and the endocrine systems. Polyurethane (TPU) is made up polyols and isocyanates and can be unhealthy to some individuals, even fatal, as it is comprised of many things, including formaldehyde and phosgene, which was used as a poisonous gas in world wars.

Some of the building materials using polyurethane are found in boards and sprayed insulation, padding of furniture and bedding, different coatings and paints, adhesives, sealants, such as wood sealers and corks, different window treatments, resin in the flooring, gaskets, and many other thermoplastics. These things, of course, exist in hospitals, usually poorly aerated.

CHAPTER 22

Bacteria

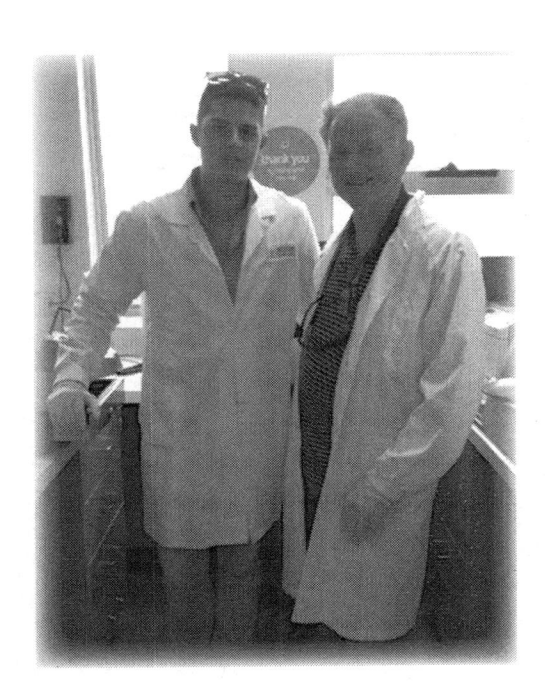

Cameron, the creator of the germ killing money drawer, and myself in the live bacteria lab.

THIS WAS A single treatment that is one activation of the closed cash drawer and its results. It should be noted that in most instances, a busy checkout person will have up to thirty customers per hour, and if that money has not been used, then it will be processed as a germ-killing venture up to fifty times an hour for possibly an eight-hour shift, or until such time as that money has all been used, increasing the killing power tremendously. It showed an activation of some 93 per cent kill rate of bacteria for a minimum one-off transaction.

The opening and closing of the cash drawer exhausts around 50 per cent of sterilized air in each drawer activation to the area around the checkout area without the use of fans and so forth, a positive reduction in airborne bacteria content. Management participation in the construction of the daily operator's float can also affect the kill rate as well as two further operations listed below.

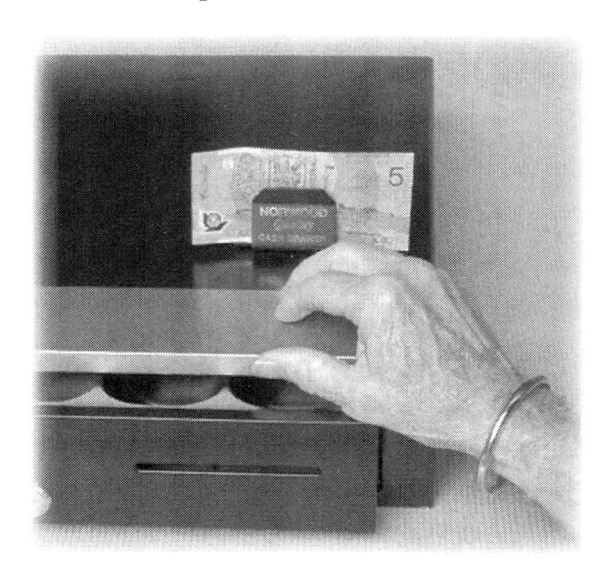

(1) *The radiation eradicator–the Parana*

The radiation eradicator is a two- to three-piece apparatus. It consists of a bill holder holding the amount tendered by the customer and given to the operator and a plate that, if used with the correct conductive bracelet, would automatically discharge any operator's electric imbalance from the right hand to the plate. Following this routine operation, the operator usually can be expected to be completely free from any static and any radiation. The cash in the drawer is sterilized and ready for the next customer, and the operation is usually radiation and static free. This technique eliminates any errors between what was tendered and the correct amount of change, giving the customer confidence in the transaction as well.

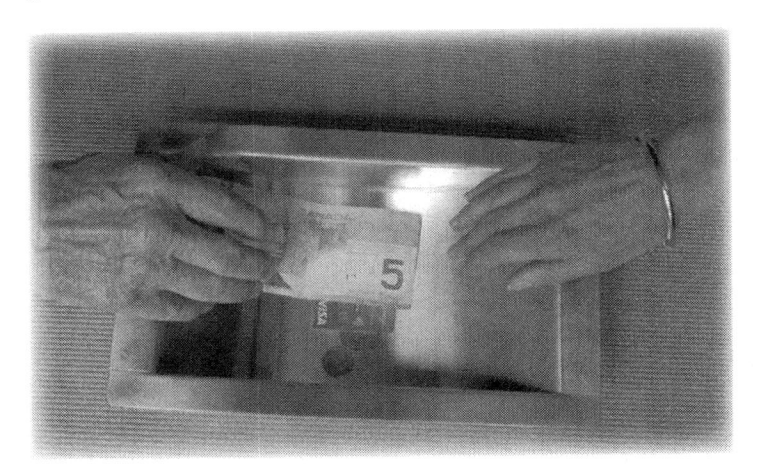

(2) *The grounding dish*

In photograph 2, you will notice that the hands never touch. The operator is on the right with the bracelet and is automatically grounded, usually eradicating any radiation content into the dish immediately. Should the receiver of the money again not touch the money or credit card and have a similar bracelet on, then he or she will be immediately safe as well. However, if the person returning the cash change does not have a bracelet, you can expect the static and radiation level, if any, to at least be reduced.

These two patented techniques go a long way towards eradicating and interchanging radical bacteria and viruses with the transfer of money. The two methods are being offered to the World Health Organization without charge in an effort to eliminate the same existing scenario happening repeatedly as it is today with credit card payments for purchases, as explained below.

Many different machines are being used in connection with the credit card industry, and the customers are so confused with all these differing machines being used to process their transactions that in the end, the tellers sometimes take the cards from the customers, and that exchange once again creates the possibility of the transfer of bacteria/viruses.

As an incentive for management to incorporate this specialized healthy drawer, you would only need one person in ten to start to look at the healthier option than currently exists. In turn, this person would encourage others to use that particular register at that particular organization. It would mean that management would have an incredible net profit by getting involved in the venture. Money talks! When compounded year after year, a 10 per cent profit adds up to a lot of money, and it would be nice to know that your staff is protected at the same time. This increase in turnover will usually come at the expense of the competitors who do not have this equipment. They would need to get involved immediately to save their clientele, the effect being that we would have a marketplace with equipment capable of destroying the diseases that surround us, both the customer and the operator.

Please note: The sale and use of this equipment is at your own risk. Full instructions on how to use the equipment safely will be supplied upon delivery, and the responsibility will be on the user of the equipment.

Richard Loyd, in his summaries of natural ways of healing, declares that there are natural ways of killing diseases. Dr. William Philpott has been using magnets as a primary and often related treatment for cancers near the surface of the body, applying them up to twenty-four hours a day. However, he points out that bipolar magnets should not be used.

As we could see on the yacht on the Caribbean, it is possible to have negative readings all the time, and it appears that they might possibly starve the positives out of the body. This may be proof that the human body, in order to survive these diseases, must not have any "feed," for the want of a better word, of increased positive content of even good body balance.

The comparative here is that Mr. Philpott is using the negative magnets to create a negative balance, whereas the policy of completing this negative balance in the body is likely to have exactly the same result but not just over a surface area. It would cost very little to have this control and could be done positively to stop the disease from progressing.

An extension of this theory is that Mr. Philpott is saying it has to be constant, twenty-four hours a day. We can go back to Albert Einstein's results with his sister and his being called Mr. Negative, referring again to the negative results on the yacht and our capacity to create an atmosphere around the body of a negative balance. It is almost as though diseases require a positive result to progress. Yes, we know it works for TB and other situations, but the way we have structured our medical profession, we expect the Western doctor to put his finger on the problem in his office. There are machines that can give negative answers, so we are in a situation where we can prevent a blowout of positives. If we get shocks on an electrical walkway this means our body is out of balance electrically and we are at risk.

Money and so forth

The banks are very much on their way to success with their hand washing techniques, but many areas still need to be improved. Perhaps like on cruise ships, a hand-sanitizing machine could be situated at the door of the bank with a friendly notice to customers: *Wash your hands before and after handling money.* A sterilizing unit should be mandatory for money coming across the counter to the teller so that money does not recirculate unsterilized.

Another way that would help is if the banks try to insist that the money they receive from the mint is *new* and not *used* and therefore germ free. Because of the fact that they have to count the money before it is dispensed, the automatic teller machines now uses notes that are new or near new–the banks should insist these machine be stocked with only *new* notes.

In Australia and Canada, our notes are plastic, which is an advantage. When they are creased, the crease remains permanent, and this too is a winning quality because it allows the UV rays to repeatedly and increasingly circulate and get around all avenues of the bacteria, including coins when placed in our germ-killing cash drawers.

On a personal level, we could set up our own system of cleansing coins by boiling them regularly and placing the sterile coins in a jar for use whenever needed. Another jar could hold those coins from your purse or pocket that have not yet gone through the process. The kids will be taking currency free from bacteria to buy their lunches and so forth. This process will stop or avoid the introduction of unrecognizable radicals creating a concoction, for want of a better word, that when mixed with their own personal bacteria will cause them to be struck down with disease.

Of course, money is not the only problem–we need to become more physical. Exercise and build up body strength. That way, you can fight off these diseases. Encourage your children to exercise instead of sitting in front of the television. When you are all sitting around the dinner table, why not ask, "Who has been for a walk today?"

Don't forget about the shoe problem, insofar as shoes being manufactured using common rubber and vinyl. There is a way of solving this. There are electrically conductive plastics and conductive rubbers which could be used in the manufacture of shoes to give us another alternative to the synthetic and rubber which we now commonly wear. This would give us constant grounding and natural body balance. It should be mandatory for manufacturers to use one or the other, making sure that all persons have electrical stability in their bodies, as they were designed to have in the creation of the human race.

While I was in Bama, I had a conversation with a woman and her husband who were going to spend three days with the centenarians some twenty minutes from the town of Bama itself, trying to learn ways to live longer. After one day, they decided to give up on the idea because of the number of annoying flies in the area, and they were departing when I left them.

While I had no trouble with the flies, nor did I have any fly problem in a Bama town personally, the Layisus would have had a similar problem because of the local effluent situation. The Hunzas were having trouble with insects in the past also, and they refused the government's offer to fumigate and eradicate the insects with poisons. The Hunzas refused to have poisons in their area because it would destroy their wine crop–they make their own wine. As a matter of interest, they created their own natural insecticide to solve the problem.

We know that flies carry disease, and disease is bacteria, but obviously this does not affect every ethnic group, and the logic of what I am going to say is pretty simple. We know that there is good and bad bacteria and that the bad bacteria can be bacteria that your body doesn't recognize. This is interesting because they can handle their own bacteria, but they cannot handle *foreign* bacteria. Their isolation restricts the amount of foreign bacteria, and this immunity to their own bacteria has been cultivated often over many hundreds of years. Although the bacteria may not be theirs personally, it is part of the bacteria recognized by their group—their neighbours are part of their ethnic group—so they automatically all have an immunity to their own local bacteria. These are local flies and insects constantly reintroducing the same bacteria amongst the group, and their isolation prevents any radicals from interfering with this historical area of bacteria.

As the reader can see, this book looks at our health from the different viewpoints of the medical world. This not only applies to Western medicine; it applies to Asian medicines as well as other medicines that exist. All have their merits, and in most instances, the people of the particular areas who use Western medicine are brainwashed by their own techniques and their own good results, but in all instances, they have had their failures. Where do we go in relation to this situation in the field of medicine, where the biggest problem that will create waves is the power of the organisations that run them and the prestige that they have achieved because of their knowledge, studies, and skills? Sufferers are living in fear because this is a different method of healing, not your conventional style that doctors are used to performing as acceptable or the "way to go" routine in our society. They need to be coaxed into looking outside the square, where they may find possible cures and alternatives. The answer is simple: the life of the person who has been diagnosed with certain death or who is going to live a miserable existence is not being considered because of the one-sided thinking of the medical profession, good intentioned as it may be. So how does the reader decide where to go? How much interest should be taken in this book as compared to other methods of medicine?

The best solution is possibly the simplest: When you have a disease, particularly a fatal disease, you ask the medico and at least one other medico what the survival rate is with the techniques or treatments that are being offered. If he is unable to offer a treatment with a good percentage success rate, look further, even if it means you have to "look outside the square."

CHAPTER 23

Eliminating Bacteria

WHETHER HE IS from overseas or from a different state or country, when a person comes into your area with rolls of notes in his pocket, he is bringing with him different bacteria. The first thing he does if he is from a different country is go to a money exchange or a bank and change his money to the local currency so he can buy food, accommodation, or whatever. That money is then passed on to a person going out of the country, taking the bacteria of that country with him. We have a continual movement of money carrying different bacteria and being transferred from one place to another.

So why hasn't it applied to these centenarians? The answer is because they do not have stores, or have very few of them, where they are transferring the various products around amongst themselves. There is a lot of bartering; you see little bags of nuts on the side of the road that come from the local nut collector. They use very little money at all. The money that they are using, of course, is usually amongst themselves—their own group. In our part of the world, we go to store checkouts where hundreds of people unknown to us have tendered money that may carry possible diseases.

Many existing cash drawers are made to a particular size and height, so designing new ones and incorporating cleansing equipment within those boundaries could be a problem.

We should all realize the number of times that coins and notes have been handled, and logic tells us that these diseases are actually being put into our pockets and our wallets. We have to get away from the old-fashioned way of handling money. As we all have to have a certain amount of cash on us, we need to know that this cash has been purified and is free from disease. This would be our counter-attack on foreign diseases spreading, and at the same time, we would be looking after our tellers and our customers.

We could just use plastic cards, right? It sounds easy, but there are disadvantages because from time to time, you need cash. For example, this would be the case if you were in a place where the taxi drivers do not accept credit cards because sometimes the costs associated with accepting cards is too great and reduces their profits—bad business. So most people put five dollars or so in their wallets for such emergencies. The big disadvantage of plastic is that people can find ways of stealing from you or from your bank account. We are giving too much information to our government regarding our financial statuses. The less the governments know about our business, the better, for they find ways of stealing from us in the end, regardless of their promises. So the solution is not plastic. The solution is to kill the viruses and bacteria on the money and credit cards.

There is a way that will positively get us out of this problem. We need to be able to keep the good viruses that our bodies can recognize and handle and destroy foreign viruses without the use of poisons, thereby creating further problems. By putting hundreds of different bacteria and/or viruses into a cash box and destroying them all at once, there would be little chance of the bacteria getting back into our wallets, as they are being repetitively cleansed—sometimes a hundred times over, and the change that is returned is completely sanitized.

I read a report put out by the Greenpeace organization on the diseases found on money. As fate would have it, I have spent a lifetime making money drawers and understand how money should be handled, so there was no person better qualified to produce something saleable, safe from governments down to unions and everyone else.

This recent study by Greenpeace was in the Asian subcontinent on currency (i.e., pounds, shillings, pence, or dollars and cents—whatever types of currency the locals were using). They did a bacteriological analysis on these notes, and 75 per cent carried contaminants with various kinds of pathogenic bacteria. They found that of the more mutilated or more used, usually the lower denomination notes, as you can image, over 44 per cent of the dirty ones had a high bacterial content. Of the currency tested, 25 per cent of the currency was considered clean. The remainder found eighteen different types of bacteria based on their colony morphology and other differentiations. Using a bacterial identification kit, I am including only five that we can identify as being serious, but as this book has pointed out already, we all vary to a great extent, so what we consider serious in one person may not be so serious in another. The idea is to have zero for both biological and electrical balance in the final analysis. The five bacteria discussed below will give the reader an idea of the seriousness of this money handling.

1. Streptococcus pyogenic (nula 1): Sometimes fatal is the golden staph. Obviously, this is something to avoid.
2. Damage to the epidermis: This skin damage is usually associated with a hospital environment. There are over thirty different variations, some having devastating effects on people who are in poor physical condition. The danger of this particular bacterium is that it prevents the medical cures from actually doing their jobs and stops the normal immune system and the medicos' efforts to

correct the bad feature of this bacterium. A better way of putting this is that it does not let your immune system function, as it should.
3. Klebsiella pneumonia: This is often found in hospitals. It is a bacterial pneumonia and is often in urinary tract infections. Pneumonia, of course, is very serious, and double pneumonia was what killed Jean's mother. This has been associated with lung diseases as well as alcoholism.
4. Salmonella: This can start a chain reaction, going from person to person, and is usually caused by bad food. If it gets associated with mycotic aneurysms, it can be fatal, and many antibiotics are proving to be unsatisfactory and unable to handle the disease. A strong immune system is your best defence against this menace. As there are so many types of this problem, immediate diagnosis in the medical world to determine exactly which type exists is essential to try to halt this disease early.
5. Enterobacter cloacae: A great extent of people have fever, most have hypotension and shock, and in about one-third of the cases, organ failure is not uncommon, with urinary tract problems sometimes difficult to fix, taking much time. This is often associated with people coming from one country to another.

We have two alternatives. One is to make sure that we don't get these diseases being transferred by the money chain. The second is to make sure that if the situation does exist, our immune systems are strong, which we can achieve by being in strong physical condition, remembering that our condition has a direct effect on the strength of our immune systems. Again, the ancients and the centenarians had few if any shops, and there was very little transference of money within their own ethnic groups. The bacterium that they handle is well established, and they can handle the bacterium that does exist within their own immune system. The bacteria just mentioned is only a fraction of the amounts that exist and rarely come in contact with them, and as such they do not have the sicknesses that we have in a civilized world. The Australian aborigines suffered to some extent from this fate, as did the North American Indians. A quick analysis of the history of these races shows that only those that have kept isolated have managed to survive. Spread of bacteria brought about by of the ease of travel nowadays is often something that the local immune system cannot recognise. Solutions need to be sought. We need to encourage those in the know to become involved in finding a way to control this spread of disease. This bypasses governments that are only concerned with how many votes they can win. This can be done at a grass-roots level to make people want to get involved for their own benefit and well-being, apart from the fact that they may or may not be one of those who is going to die from one of these dreadful diseases. These diseases are caused by civilization, and the spreading of disease by circulating money is one of the big problems.

These are just a few of the many bacteria, viruses that were found by Greenpeace in their investigations, and we intend to do a study on the fact that the Australia notes are made with plastic; we can then get a full overview that exists between plastic and paper money.

We apologise at this point for including the medical world in our world of physics. However, with the use of physics, we will endeavour to stop the progressions of diseases with the view of our living trouble-free and disease-free lives. This solution is available and will be shown in the conclusions towards the end of this book.

Counter-attack

With the information that we have and the way we found it, starting back with the centenarians, it would have to be considered a tremendous amount of luck or fate that this information was found in this particular method because the answer is still to come. It started when Greenpeace did their study in the Asian subcontinent on the danger of bacteria on money, notes, and coins.

Greenpeace showed us how we were actually getting these diseases by the transference of money. We know from what we have just studied that foreign bacteria—that is, bacteria that we are not equipped to personally handle or recognize—is what our immune systems cannot handle. The solution to is to *kill the bacterium that is* being transferred on the money itself.

Working with Cameron Taylor, we were both blessed by the fact that we have no medical knowledge; everything would be based on the principle of physics. We had the information and decided to create a solution to the problem. The problem being the constant attack by viruses through the money and credit card system. We couldn't change it overall, but we could change the method of destroying the bacteria in both of those systems. The problem with this is that the inventions have to be such that this equipment is used and is viable economically to a standard that achieves the purpose. The point is to eradicate radicals that are being introduced into particular localized areas. The overall principal would be to make an invisible cage that by both technique and design could achieve a protective area around the checkout department of every store, big or small, in the cash-handling section. The idea is to protect the persons that are involved in cash or credit card transactions, including the customer and the operator of the machine, with the result of improved sterilized air in the area and virus/bacteria elimination.

To make the operation from the point of view of manufacturing economical, it is necessary to have the proprietors of the equipment onside. The government can help here by declaring the principal cost of the equipment as tax deductible. In Australia, anything to do with business is tax deductible. The cost of the equipment comes off the profit level at the end, and you pay taxes on the balance. So it does not really matter how much it costs, for this deduction is transferred over years and the businessperson is in fact getting this cost/outlay back over a period of time. If that facility does not exist in particular countries, then it might be suggested by the business community that it should be considering the savings from the point of view of health, which the government is involved in. It is a major cost but remember if the diseases are reduced then so will the sick days. If a person is seriously ill perhaps terminal then it is not likely that they would be working, which means he or she is not paying taxes—not good business for the government. The idea is to make this bacteria-destroying money drawer or tray in a consistent size or alternatively organize it in such a way that it becomes a totally incarcerated and controlled germ-killing device within the allotted space. This technique, while being invisible to both the operator and the customer, has an indicator showing the customer that the product is in operation, destroying the bacteria and so forth. The purpose of this is to encourage the customer to come back, knowing someone has looked after him from a health point of view. This would also create a new customer base against his competitors. This is just good business and good health.

The statistics below will give you an idea of what Cameron and I achieved with our invention: a money drawer that kills germs without the use of chemicals and the operating techniques that go with it to expand on this system and utilize the information that we have remembered going back as far as Bama in China.

These statistics from Greenpeace Investigations give you only a fraction of the idea. Only five of the samples were examined. That gives the overall picture of the disaster. This together with the results from our own live experiments and goodness only knows what we might finish up with in hospital.

These techniques are safe for people, but if any operator feels unhappy physically in using the equipment, it can be immediately turned off to stop any complications. With every unit, instructions are enclosed. It will be the responsibility of the shop owner to explain to the customer that the machine is killing any bacteria on the money to protect them and everyone else they serve over the counter.

It is obvious that we have to verify the impact of what we have invented, and we are going to apply this to Australian currency. We have treated money using the sterilising drawer system which we have manufactured. Australian notes are plastic, so we have also used the same system for overseas paper money to make sure that all avenues are covered worldwide. The results were impressive and are recorded below.

Official Analysis/Findings

Project Number		
Sample Number	E13/007206-001	E13/007206-003
Client Reference	Sampled 15/4/13	Sampled 15/4/13

Description	Australia Pre-UV	Australia Post-UV
Staphylocc=occus (COAG+VE) (GWFB 4.1)	72000 CFU/G	5000 CFU/G
E. Coli (GWFB 6.7)	120000 CFU/Swab	4800 CFU/Swab
Plate Count (GWFB 1.1)	290000 CFU/G	21000 CFU/G
Mould Count (GWFB 2.1)	<100 CFU/G	<100 CFU/G
Yeast Count (GWFB 2.1)	2100 CFU/G	<100 CFU/G

NATA Accredited Approval No. 1619

Richard Loyd Phd comment: *The dealing and killing of mould can make the difference between life and death.*

Everyday Language–Eradication

Staphylococcus	72000	5000	93.06%
E.coli	120000	4800	96%
Plate count	290000	21000	92.76%
Mould Count	<100	<100	0–100%

CHAPTER 24

Recommendations and Solutions

WE WILL BE setting up a website, and as these different anti-static and anti-radiation inventions are proven to our satisfaction, we will brand them so that you will see that we have actually tested them and that they are not just open to opportunists who don't care about you personally and are only interested in making money. On the website, you will get reasonable assurance that they will actually work for you.

Extensive studies by brilliant people have shown that electromagnetic radiation is exactly what it sounds like– it is about electricity, which is positive and negative.

Of course, this brings forward the concept that mobile phones are possibly involved because of the increase in cancers and other diseases which is positively verified as true, and the research is quite brilliant. Dr. Peter Finch and his research team have shown that using a mobile phone for an hour a day showed changes in cell growth, particularly the male cell, which plays an important role in an improved immune system—and that is, of course, what we are talking about. Namely, that we get our immune systems built up by a supply of energy over and above the normal energy required every day.

We have to understand that we cannot change the weeping power lines around and that mobile phones are dangerous. We don't like the idea of radio towers being beside us. There are so many things that we don't know, but there are things we do know, and these things we *can* beat. I am going to offer solutions. Hopefully we might get governments onside but normally, until it affects their voting power, Nothing happens. The solutions that I am going to offer—as far as feasibility—will be totally natural, so there should not be any worries unless there is something unusual about the person who is going to use these products and devices that I am going to put forward to you. An on/off switch often solves this scenario.

The only way that you or I can survive is to attempt to solve the problems personally. Because we all vary in our lives, our works also vary, and we must anticipate our daily activities in relation to staying alive. It is all down now to a personal level. The fact is that civilization has created one giant killing machine insofar as electrics in our bodies. All parts of our bodies are electric machines.

People with cancer often cannot understand how they got it. So how does it actually get inside these people? Why is it so desperately dangerous, and why doesn't dilution with plenty of air necessarily solve the problem?

Don't forget that my mum recommended using Epsom salts or its equivalent every month for cleaning out anything caught in the bowels, the colon, or the intestines. If you are being treated by any of the various treatments for cancer relief, then formaldehyde or any catalyst that can have the effect of promoting your disease, such as cancer, can remain inside your body, recharging your disease constantly unless you get rid of it—dispose of it. Simple logic tells you this.

Some specialists who go by the book might say that it is unnatural to use such a product as Epsom salts. It might be too much of a shock on your body because the result is quite extreme. It might be considered unnatural, but so is disease. I suggest that you discuss with your medical doctor this usage of a small dose of Epsom salts: usually 1 dessertspoon (ten milligrams) in warm water to dissolve it. Drinkable Epsom salts (also known as magnesium sulphate) are available from chemists and are incorporated into three-fourths of a teacup of warm water, or approximately ten milligrams for a person five feet ten inches and weighing approximately seventy-five kilos. When cooled off and dissolved, drink a few quick gulps and then drink plenty of water afterwards. The result, as mentioned before, is quite dramatic, and you will need plenty of time on the toilet to dispose of any catalyst that is likely to mix with bacteria within the body.

Let's take it from another specialist. Dr. Richard Loyd, PhD, wrote an article called "Improving Health of Cancer Patients" (from July 16, 2010), wherein it says to remove toxins—and I am assuming that we are calling formaldehyde a toxin—he says to use an herbal mixture that contains bugle weed, such as Metal Release. Platinum Plus Essential Amino Acids to remove the toxins. Using three times a day on an empty stomach along with a good multivitamin can enable your body to make the proteins that the body uses to carry toxic metals away.

So you have two known alternatives, including one of my own remedies that I can vouch for. I am still here, and Mum made 104; moreover, it is quick, but the decision has to be yours alone. You might find that your physician suggests the reintroduction of other good bacteria into your body at a time soon after using either of those two options.

With serious diseases such as cancer, it should be noted that there has to be at least one other catalyst to pick up the remaining 15 per cent possible contaminant. It will be interesting to note the situation if we can eliminate 100 per cent by finding out what that other 15 per cent is made up of.

It should also be noted that various catalysts, when mixed with our own personal bacteria, together with the man-made poisons, create your own personal disease as a result of your activities. Again, the idea is to try to clean out the catalysts and poisons.

Formaldehyde or any catalyst that can have the effect of promoting your disease, such as cancer, can remain inside your body, recharging the disease constantly. Simple logic tells you that unless you get rid of this catalyst, it is likely to mix with bacteria within the body and therefore must be disposed of.

We can take a further extension of the episode on the yacht. Again, everybody was showing minus answers in relation to the positive and negative results that were available. Let's go one step further and visualize a possibility, and this is strictly a possibility. Let's assume that some people have or have had a disease, and let's assume that they are bombarded with negative ions. Is it possible that we can actually starve those positive results or, putting it differently, is it perhaps necessary to have a supply of positive ions for diseases to survive? It is almost as though this particular feature in the body is feeding them. The goal is to finish with a minus zero balance. It's a strong argument that a zero balance stops diseases from growing–the disease requires an imbalance to progress, and it can be "held off" with balance.

It would cost a fraction of the money involved to treat people who are prepared to get involved without chemotherapy and the poisons around them, isolating them and supplying them with a constant barrage of negative ions. We may even have the simplest cure looking at us and we don't even recognize it, as we are assuming that the solution has to be medical. It does not have to be medical. It wasn't medical for Mr. Einstein's sister–it's initially a matter of historical cultivated physics.

Considering and re-examining past medical experiments that have been conducted and/or requested, they may not have taken into account the importance of the electrical body-balancing feature being instituted before, during, and after the experiments.

CHAPTER 25

A Miracle? Positive Verification 2013

I AM CONFIDENT that I am on the right track, and if this track cannot be disproved, then the entire book is valuable. So many people are dying around me from these diseases, and I am hopeful that I will get the message through to the general public as well as these people at risk. I have spent over a year researching and studying, and then a particular incident occurred …

Situated between Sydney, in New South Wales, and Brisbane, the capital of the state of Queensland, is a small town known as Mullumbimby. The town is set against the magnificent backdrop of Mount Chincogan and the famous Mount Warning. It is touted as the "biggest little town in Australia." As with all the centenarian towns, the main highway bypasses the town, which has the reputation of being one of the best places to live in Australia. It has won an award for being the cleanest. There are two main streets, each only being approximately one hundred yards long, and behind these streets is a small mountain range.

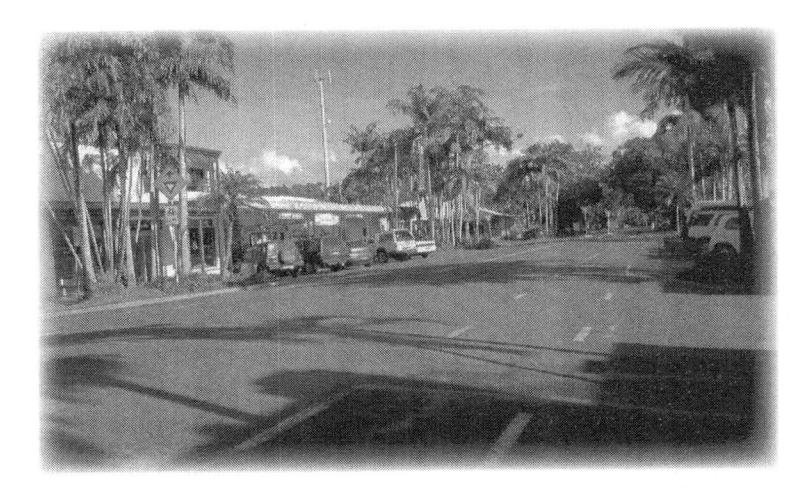

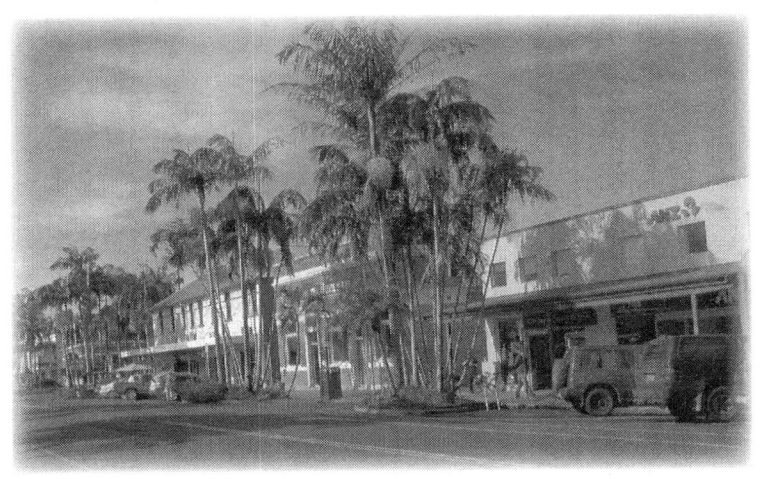

Mullumbimby

My brother's widowed wife, Beth, lives in this beautiful little town, about halfway down a hill protected from the southerly trade winds. There is a creek below the house, and in the distance is the beautiful Brunswick River. Any trade winds from the north-east feed the town with clean air.

Because the town is small, there is much camaraderie, not unlike the centenarians. Big crowds go to the local football games and watch their children growing up happily. There appears to be little disease, and they have a good little school, hospital, golf course, and so forth. Everybody considers it a nice place to live.

Unfortunately, Beth has had lung cancer for some years, and the situation has been very serious, to the extent that in the past she has had to use a large metal Oxy Care machine within the house, thus making her life inactive and restricted. She does crochet as a hobby, and she does it beautifully. We feel that the radicals that were associated with her disease, as with all diseases, being bacteria or viruses as the principal content, was likely caught in town, when she was working in a hospital environment. Smoking no doubt caused the lung cancer, as she was a heavy smoker for most of her life, and even though she knew the problems associated with smoking (as her occupation was that of a qualified nurse), she still continues with the habit, although it is now reduced to two cigarettes per day.

Because of the repetitiveness of her hobby of crocheting, she has carpel tunnel syndrome affecting the usefulness of her hands, making money handling difficult. Her son, a widower because of a tragic accident, lives with her and does most of the shopping. For the pain, she had been on regular doses of morphine. The morphine was in the form of patches supplied by her medical practitioner and posted to her. The only other form of relief was strong Panadol. Because she had very little sun, she took a daily dose of Vitamin D.

Some years ago, she agreed to try pranic healing. She had had only one treatment of chemotherapy and did not continue. She had one session of pranic healing, and that night she had to be hospitalized, even though she was never actually touched by the hands of the healer! This healing was a crystal healing, almost identical to what Master Danny performed on Jean, and Jean's only reaction was a giant clean out of her bowels and of her intestines. Of course, the diseases were different; one was a giant melanoma and the other lung cancer. When Beth came out of hospital, she was marginally improved. Today she uses the oxygen twice a day, once going to bed and once in the morning. There has been slow improvement.

Now, as a reader, I want you to relate this back to the centenarians, the Einsteins, the Okinawans, and the circumstances that existed with the illness and our efforts to help Jean. Of course, there was also the isolation from civilization and many other parallels.

In December 2013, I rang Beth to wish her Merry Christmas. She asked if I had heard the news. I replied, "No, what is it?" She said that the doctors had done tests on her, and the cancer had disappeared. They were calling it a miracle! Beth said she had been told that she still had scarring. The doctors don't know what will happen with that or if the cancer will come back in another form, but the important thing is that *the cancer is no longer there*! Comprehensive documentation is available to the medical world.

It certainly was a merry Christmas for Beth. I feel we are very close to a cure. Now let's look at what happened to Beth—the bad luck in relation to her hand, which has compounded her immobility, causing isolation in her lifestyle. Beth was isolated from the general public due to her health situation, living in a small town with very little road traffic, thus eliminating lots of airborne bacteria. Her home is almost identical to that of Jean's except hers is brick and Jean's was timber. Both homes are more than twenty years old, and therefore any poisons/pollutants used in their construction would have dissipated many years ago.

The home is on the hill going down to the water, which in Beth's case is a river and Jean's is a bay, with improved negative ion content. Beth cannot handle money due to the carpal tunnel affecting the hands, and my mum was losing her sight, which affected her mobility, causing personal isolation, and she could not handle money either! Neither of them could shop, so they were not at risk within a store situation, where every transaction can cause a person to be infected/reinfected with a number of various bacteria or diseases.

You can use the workable features—be it one or all—that suit your lifestyle and medical condition. Even if you consider yourself to be in good physical shape and refer them not only to where cancers are concerned but to most diseases, just remember that we all vary Individually and what may suit one person may not suit another. If in doubt, consider what is natural or what was natural thousands of years ago, before we interfered with nature and changing lifestyles.

There will be additions not only from myself but also from other people who have experienced miracles and are reading this book. With their help and with the use of our website, we can improve the power of this book and its capacity to heal to a greater extent than it is being represented here.

To the millions of people who are looking for an alternative, you can use Beth, Jean, my 104-year-old mum, the centenarians, and Albert Einstein as examples. You will notice the similarities throughout the book. Quote them and these now-known methods and successes that extended their lives. Are we close to a cure? *Are we actually there now?*

Thank you, Beth, for the verification—and to all those who have been involved in the production of this book, I extend my thanks as well. An invitation exists by the writer to disprove the accuracy of any of this information, and if it cannot be disproved, then a cure likely exists today.

The beauty of this book is that it can be used individually or with the help of a dedicated government, such as the government of Brazil, which financed the radiation experiment, or big business (e.g., the manufacture of thousands of Kirlian machines, the germ-killing cash drawers already in initial production; the Winky shield, protecting women's breasts and those women who are pregnant; and so on). Note that t'ai chi is a powerful technique and should only be performed twice a day unless under the supervision of a specialist in that area of exercise.

So we have a situation within my own family of two miracles occurring, neither of which is blood related. One was the extended life, in near perfect condition, of Jean;

the other is Beth being informed of the giant improvement in her health because of the cancer disappearing.

At this moment, let's try to understand what the word miracle means. A miracle is something that you cannot understand or comprehend. If you can understand and know what has happened, then it is not a miracle. The contents of this book explain exactly what occurred and how the illnesses were controlled, often inadvertently. Because of Beth's condition, she walked around the house with bare feet, and only when things got cold did she wear socks, thus giving her a positive grounding effect nearly 100 per cent of the time.

Beth's unfortunate and disappointing physical condition and then her recovery create an interesting scenario that warrants investigation. We know that isolation from the Western world was a benefit in fighting her disease.

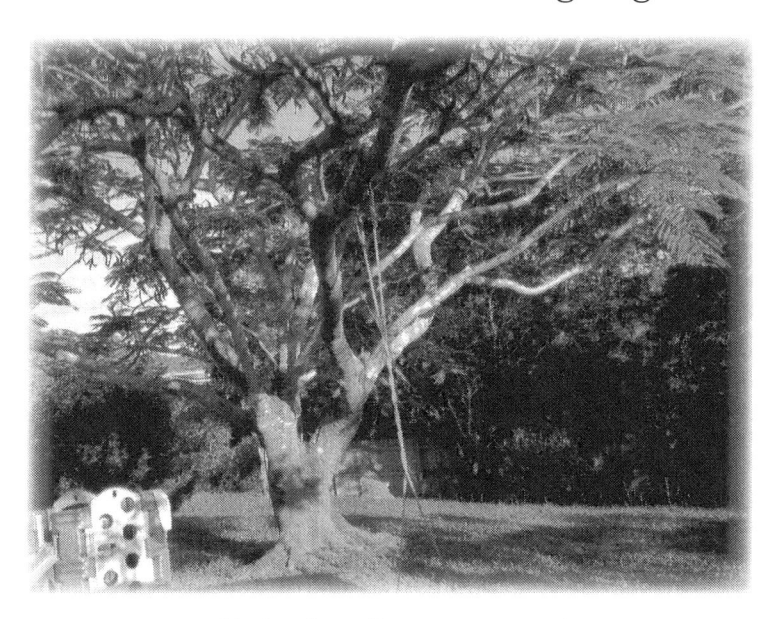

Beth's backyard–trees everywhere

Beth smoked, but she cut back on her smoking dramatically; nevertheless, the fact remains that she did get cancer, so as well as the nicotine catalyst and/or the affects from cigarette smoke, she must have been or must be carrying some other igniting ingredient for the cancer to develop. This catalyst or the contributing factor must have been removed for the disease to actually disappear. We may never know what concoction, ingredient, or bacteria actually caused the disease, but what is conclusive is that they were reduced to such an extent that the cancer could not survive, even though Beth was occasionally still inflicting the nicotine catalyst into her body.

Then a breakthrough

Feeling that there is some form of missing link at this particular point, I elected to fly to the Gold Coast, hire a car, take my electronic equipment with me, and test Beth in regard to her location. I was greeted warmly. Upon arrival, I found that the whole family was there to greet me, including the grandchildren, and we had a very happy night. Beth put me up for the night, and we had some nice long-overdue time together.

When most of them left, I asked Helen, Dale, Beth, and Mark if they would mind if I hooked electrical equipment up to them, and they all hesitated, although they showed great interest, as you would expect. As I did with the centenarians I had tested, I showed what it came up to. I myself came up with a great negative answer, which pleased me, of course: it was -.2 of a volt.

This probably could not have been better–similar to what my reading was on the yacht. I then put the machine on each of them, and the machine showed a surprising result individually, almost identical in each case of two-thousand-odd negative volts. This was extreme, and the last time this happened was when I got the giant results in Okinawa, and then I thought the batteries were faulty and we went hunting for batteries. But when I came back to test that woman in Okinawa, she came up with a normal zero number.

Concerned about this result, I asked Dale if she would come down to the town with me, where I would test her away from the house. We went to a park that was isolated from council wiring, and Dale's result came up at -.2 volts, a perfect result, the same as my reading in the house. I measured myself and came up with a similar negative answer again. We went to another part of the town and came up again with good negative answers, just like on the yacht, which is an indication that the town is an area literally fully of negative ions, giving you negative balances all the time. This is obviously an impressive place to live, but what happened with that giant negative answer we got in Beth's home? I was totally confused, as it was as though the house itself was overwhelmingly negative for some reason, having an effect on the situation in or around the home itself. I feel that the results I recorded at Beth's home previously were excessive because I had just arrived in town and had not had time to acclimatise, unlike the others in the room. My mind flashed to Einstein and how he could boast of getting excesses of negative ions needed to cure his sister.

Confused in my own mind as to what was happened, I started to think about the Chinese method of curing people. They don't dot the i's and cross the t's but if something works, they record it and continue to use it if it doesn't do you any harm. The idea of feng shui is that they don't know why it works, but they have people who go into other people's homes and say that it's a good home to buy or that it's better than another location because of the feng shui feelings that these so-called experts get. Let's just assume now—and I am absolutely going to prove that this is right—that that feeling of well-being that they get in an area where you have an excessive amount of negative ions does exist. In other words, we are explaining the physics of negative ions in particular locations and particular rooms, and these negative ions ensure that you are not getting any positive effects, which we know are no good in relation to our electrical body balance. Such as we had on the boat, they offer additional strength and energy to combat disease. We were jumping out of our skins—everyone in that room was laughing and happy.

When I left Beth, I came back to Sydney and tried to analyse what had happened. All these people were locals in the room. My reading was different from theirs, but then again, there are millions of plusses and minuses in the body and it is logical to assume that it takes time to develop a strengthened balance that is no excess of positives. Feeling that I had been left up in the air and not being totally confident on April 14, 2014—which was two weeks after my first meeting with the family—I hopped in my car, taking another independent person, whom I'll call Edward (not his real name), with me, and drove up to the Gold Coast and Mullumbimby and redid the readings.

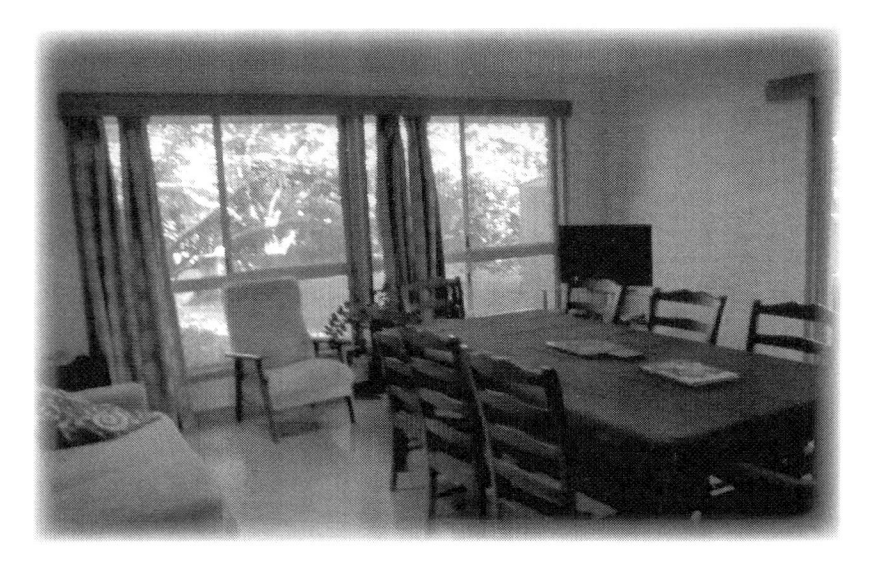

Main feng shui room

This now gets interesting because we can work a *cure* around this. Readings on April 1 came up with my measuring two volts, and everyone else's readings were within one hundred volts, up to 2,300 negative. After driving up there almost two weeks later, I came up with -0 as a reading, Beth was -2,300 again, Mark came up with -1,257, and Edward came up -1. So we have the family members' readings with tremendous minus situations and absolutely no positives, which we should not have in our bodies anyway, except as a balance against the negative. We then went down to town again, and I came up with a beautiful -2 volt reading again.

On our second trip, Beth came up with -2, Mark came up with -601, I came up with -3, and Edward came up with -10. This was nothing like the first time, where we had all these excessive amounts of negative answers, and the situation appears to be the difference in the climate at the time. In the first instance, on April 1, we had had a very dry period, one of the driest for some years, and then prior to our arriving, we had a dramatic downpour of rain, and in that downpour, the temperature was twenty-six degrees, which is enough to create evaporation. We now have to remember that Mr. Einstein concluded that evaporation is the cause of negative ions. Being on the side of the hill, full of trees and all the non-poisonous features that go with an aged home, is why we had that excess of negative ions. It appears that according to Mr. Einstein's theory, we cannot have too many negative ions—he talked of it as being a health feature. That is why we had that overload of negative ions in the first instance, and in the second instance, we had come into a situation where the temperature was nineteen degrees maximum on April 14 and there was absolutely no wind. It was a very still location. We had a situation where the climate could affect the amount of evaporation and the creation of negative ions to extreme levels, and this is how Beth was cured, by being in a location in a town that even when things were dry and quiet, you were still getting negative answers. It improves the theory that we should not have any excessive positives ions in our bodies at all. There should be no more than a zero–a perfect balance.

In the second location, we had virtually no atmospheric activity at all. We can create any volume of negative ions we want to defeat disease, not just cancer. So as part of the concoction/cocktail that we possess, we can include the creation of negative ions as part of our destroying effect of disease. The elimination of our concoction a piece at a time virtually prevents the disease from continuing, as happened with Jean, and if we can eradicate the other factors in our personal cocktails, then we can win our personal struggle–the individual war being carried on within our own bodies. If we don't have these locations, then we can mechanically make this equipment. It exists today, and it can create body balance, kill germs, and prevent static and its accumulative effect. We can also control the climate in confined areas–that is, when we can't defend ourselves against civilization and the problems that come with it.

I believe that Jean was poisoned by civilization. In fact, I feel that the bacteria or viruses were probably a result of her constant travelling and contact with different ethnic groups–often personally ungrounded.

As an act of sincere love, I made a promise to Jean to try to find out what made the melanoma develop. I have done the very best I can, but I still wish I could have done more at the time. Jean was the love of my life, and I failed to stop the cancer, even though it was halted for years, with her being in perfect condition because we thought outside the conventional medical square that we are all involved in in the Western world. When the disease was in remission, we should have duplicated all our efforts that got her to the point of living longer than doctors predicted and pulling off what the medical profession called a miracle.

Could I have done any better or any more? The answer is no. I did not have the information that I have now. We know we must regularly clean out our systems in the hope that we rid our bodies of these igniters/concoctions, and I feel this is a very important factor.

You have been given the guidelines here. Try to apply the principles. It is obvious that civilization is the cause of the spread of disease. We need to copy what the centenarians do. Isolate yourself when possible, sail around the world, do the same thing repeatedly, play sports, live a good healthy lifestyle. Follow the book and prevent disease, and if you are unlucky enough to get any of these dreadful illnesses, consider all the suggestions contained herein and apply them as closely as you possibly can in your everyday life.

Live, love, laugh, be happy, be a centenarian, and only look as if you are sixty-five years old!

CHAPTER 26

Conclusion

FAMILY AND FRIENDS often asked me why I am doing all this research now that Jean has passed away. I told them of my promise to Jean, that I would find a solution with my inventions to prevent other people from ending up in her situation. I think about what we did without having any medical knowledge, the research and inventions giving me a full picture of the life and death of Jean and the miracle of this extended life and how it came to be so long, and the question is, what more could I have done?

It is obvious that we all carry a huge volume of bacteria, and somehow Jean's must have had a catalyst that reacted with some of these bacteria to such an extent that it got out of control, thereby creating a melanoma.

Jean tried to help herself by taking high volumes of health and vitamin supplements to boost her energy and support her system. She saw the pranic specialist, who had the capacity of cleansing the carcinogenic content from her body.

It must be appreciated that this pranic system of health is not just the ability to remove and clean your personal plumbing system. It requires major study and is beyond my explanations. We are hoping that this book will give people in a serious situation a reprieve in the form of extended life in good condition. So we don't want to assume that this is the only possibility that this pranic medicine has—this different creation of energy. Also, had I had the knowledge of the handling of metal and the capacity we now have of transferring electrical charges out of the body in the interest of creating normal balance, then I believe we could had extended Jean's life even further.

The money from the cash register drawers (again, our new one will be called the Parana—Parana being the aggressor to germs and viruses) could have contributed to the bacteria/viruses that Jean may have unknowingly acquired.

We have to be thankful for that woman on the hill in Okinawa regarding that situation of metal in a controlled personal electrical situation. We have proved that the control of radiation and static are related to a certain extent. Both are unnatural and should not be found in the human body in a modern civilized world. Within the book, a solution exists for this as well. Remember the woman in Okinawa with the thick headgear and clothing, which I thought was to prevent snakebite? It would have had a degree of radiation protection in that particular situation.

I feel that possibly what happened in Jean's case was that the melanoma was not being fed (due to the positive or excess of negative ions) because of her lifestyle and the constant walking, which created energy and helped her greatly, so in the end, maybe it was a reoccurrence of the carcinogenic bacteria that was let out of its controlled cage, for want of a better explanation, thereby killing her.

I wonder as I write this if it should be a standard procedure for people with these diseases to regularly cleanse their whole internal system as Jean did, perhaps once a year or whatever the doctors think is not too much of a personal shock to the system, keeping any catalyst from mixing with the bacteria.

Had I had the opportunity to do it over again, we possibly would have done that every year. From personal experience, there would be no more dramatic reactions from it, as were my experiences with my mum.

Jean may have had some of these unhealthy ingredients in her system for possibly years. Cancer was around thousands of years ago, as verified by Marcus Aurelius around 160 AD, although years ago, it may not have been know by the name of cancer, as we know it today. He was co-emperor of Rome and had to supervise the army and the conquered areas of the Roman Empire. There was the situation where various bacteria were introduced, which was totally unnatural to both the conqueror and the conquered. This may have been why many empires disappeared over time, with the introduction of foreigners and what they carry with them.

To the question of where do we go from here, the electrical balance has to be twenty-four hours a day; this is to give you the energy and the strength to fight off these diseases. The biggest problem with body balance I have found is in the bedroom, and other researchers have found the same problem—that it is difficult to get down to a perfect balance during your sleeping hours.

We know that having negative ions allows us to get back into balance, but this does not appear to be helping in the bedroom situation at all, giving rise to the possibility that we can be at risk, although unlikely because of the location, but it prevents the introduction of perfect body balance. We must not forget that Mr. Einstein and his associates designed machines that actually manufacture negative ions. These are in the marketplace, and they could be used in the bedroom to perhaps balance this situation. Hospitals that are usually poorly ventilated could use this equipment immediately.

This balance is important; we need to keep our bodies in balance 100 per cent of the time. We may have already found cures to all diseases simply by following the basics of this book. Whether it is practical to be jumping out of our skins with negative ions, as we were on the yacht, is still debatable.

In the effort to meet my commitment and give readers solutions to their problems, we need to appreciate that this does not have to end with these solutions. The biggest problem has been man-made electricity and the problem of rubber grounding the feet. What has not been discussed in detail is the principal of yin and yang, the ancients' methods of healing going back to Tibetan theories and so forth. Yin and yang, including the elimination of stress to reduce this imbalance, has a lot to do with body balance, but theories of yin and yang go back to before electricity was created, so there are obviously other methods of achieving body balance. When we analyse the food of the centenarians and the long-lived, we realize that there is often a big discrepancy of acid and alkali in the food chain. Should we be able to correct that as only one of the yin and yang methods of balance and then add that to what we have learnt from the experiences in this book, then we can increase our bodies' stability and energy to try to carry out the lifestyles and the modern ways of the current world we live in … immediately.

Integration

The biggest problem we have is that although we have this information, we are totally brainwashed in our thinking that the solution must be made by the medical profession. They are so very strong and so very powerful that nothing else is considered possible. Next week we will hear another breakthrough that the medical profession has worked out, and there is no denying that they are brilliant and will eventually, particularly with this information of body balance, get a solution, as they have boasted about doing within twenty years.

The thing that is wrong with the medical profession's theory is that they are trying to cure diseases, but they could anticipate these diseases before they take hold, with the use of Karlian photography, as mentioned previously. If we can only get the medical profession with all their skills together and *integrate* some of these alternate medicines, including what we have written in this book ... A person may go to the doctor with, say, a common cold, but whilst he is there, if they had a Karlian machine in their surgery or waiting room, then the person could have an image taken and give it to his or her physician. This may uncover a problem with the liver, bowel, or what have you. Doctors may charge a nominal fee or incorporate it with their scheduled charge—or may even have a coin-operated machine.

In fact, they could have a star on the door of the surgery, indicting to a perspective patient coming in that this surgery offers a better overview of their health, and from the doctors' point of view, it would give them more stability within their own patients and practice. So when we get this Karlian machine in operation and in volume, you can then see for yourself the overall picture of your health.

The dangers to us all are two things:

1. Don't just read this book and shelve it. It costs you so little to be involved, just by being aware of the situation and the risk that we are all in.

2. Don't be too lazy to make the regular effort of looking after yourself. Some people say that if you live you live and if you die you die, but you have to consider your family. They are going to miss you, and you are not doing the right thing by them by not looking after yourself.

All the basics are here to give you an extended life. The Roman Empire failed because the population got too soft. You will notice the comparison as you walk along the street of the people of our civilized world. The conditions are not unlike the failure of the Roman Empire. We need to be part of this medical survival–wake up, get up, and walk! It is up to each of us.

My experience as I have written this book has shown that when people had diseases such as Parkinson's disease and other diseases and I put the equipment on them, they were showing perfect balance, which means that the positives and negatives were equal–their yin and their yang. However, if the energy source was the good negative and they are actually accumulating the energy as we had on the boat, then we feel that this stored energy should have helped to prevent any disease in the first instance. Then can we starve the progress, which we have proved we can do, to such an extent that the energy source is greater than the disease? If so, how to do it?

It should not be forgotten that Mr. Hansell and Mr. Einstein had the capacity to manufacture negative ions to extents exceeding 100 per cent at that time.

We are talking about the early 1920s. I have seen no instance of people in these various diseases switching on machines to increase the amount of negative ions that are necessary to give you this additional energy. It is almost as thought this additional energy capacity has been totally overlooked, possibly because it wasn't thought of in the world of medicine. We are looking at this from the point of view of physics on the body.

I feel a new chapter has been written regarding the treatment of cancer and diseases once this book's information and procedures are taken into account.

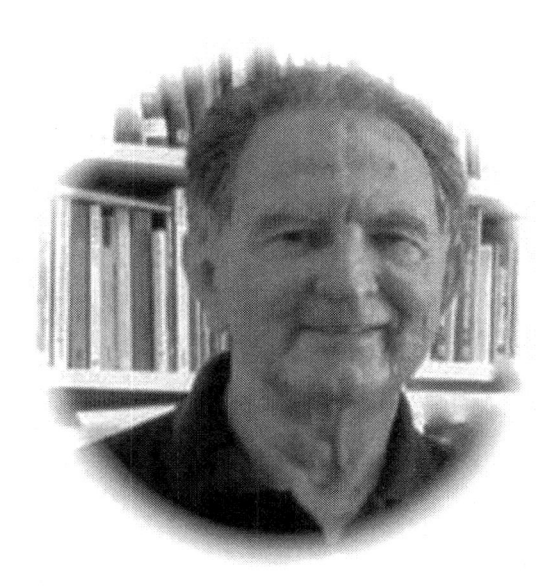

Don Wood, Author

Don Wood is a family man with four daughters and five grandchildren. He has a family-operated business in Sydney, Australia.

Don was a champion athlete. He is a current World Masters champion in the yachting field, and his yachting adventures have taken him to all the oceans of the world, including Cape Horn–short-handedly. He played rugby and soccer, and he is a self-confessed golf hacker. Whilst completing his army service, he was what was known in those days as a welterweight boxing champion. He raced catamarans worldwide representing Australia. He and his wife, Jean, loved life!

He had previously had success in inventing, and this turned out to be invaluable as he attempted to find a nonmedical solution to give to the world an alternative solution in the treatment of cancer. In his world travels, he got to understand different ethnic groups and their approach to handling health problems.

His life was shattered by the news that his beloved wife was diagnosed with a terminal liver melanoma. He made a promise to Jean, and having no medical knowledge, he set out to find alternative treatments for the terrible disease of cancer.

Source and references used throughout the book:

Richard Loyd, PhD, "Improving Health of Cancer Patients; *The Okinawa Program*, William J. Beaty; Static Electricity Means Voltage, The Mediterranean Solution smh.com.au/lifestyle/e/diet- and-fitness/Mediterranean-diet-cuts-risk-of-first- heart attack, Paavo Airóla, PhD; Ramon Estruch of the University of Barcelona; Greenpeace; the International Agency for Research on Cancer; *The Crystal Bible*, by Judy Hall; Phillip Nintschke; Corbis Corporation; Bridget Waterhouse, Jason Waterhouse, Ben, Sam Lay, Ben Bolenski, John Dumay, "Power Lines – Not Radiation but Static Electricity Causes Disease and Cancer," by Peter Staheli.

Miracles

Do you believe in miracles?

Where there is a cure of a serious disease using natural remedies that are outside the medical profession's ways, surely this would have to be classed as a miracle.

Read the book and apply the suggestions—and perhaps you too can experience a miracle.

Don

www.beatingcancerwitheinstein.com